CONTAINS RECYCLED PARTS

My Triple Organ Transplant Journey
and the Science of Gratitude

AIMÉE MACKOVIC

For information about this title or to order other books and/or electronic media, contact the publisher:

Two Sisters Writing & Publishing®

TwoSistersWriting.com

18530 Mack Avenue, Suite 166

Grosse Pointe Farms, MI 48236

ISBN   978-1-956879-48-3 (Hardcover)

ISBN   978-1-956879-49-0 (Paperback)

ISBN   978-1-956879-50-6 (eBook)

Printed in the United States of America

All the stories in this work are true.

Cover and Graphic Design: Illumination Graphics.

Cover artwork by Tara Thelen.

Author photos: The Mackovic Family Collection.

For K, my heart and liver donor

"There are good days and there are bad days, and this is one of them."

— Lawrence Welk

"You can watch if you want. I'm going to play until the end of this life."

— Gabrielle Zevin

Author

Tomorrow and Tomorrow and Tomorrow

Contents

ONE

I HAVE ALMOST DIED AT LEAST TWICE.

The first time I almost died, I am three years old. My mother and Aunt Joanie are leaving to go shopping for groceries and such. As the keys are in the ignition, the babysitter runs out to the garage, flushed with panic, holding me in her arms. I am turning blue and not breathing. Without thinking, my mother takes me by my feet, turns me upside down, and thwack! After a few swift pats on the back, I spit out a cherry Life Saver. Seemingly unaware of my imminent brush with death, I pick up the Life Saver and pop it back into my mouth. The second time I almost died . . . well, that is where this story begins. Grab your beverage and snack of choice and buckle up.

I suggest whisky.

TWO

THE BIRTHSTONE OF MARCH IS THE AQUAMARINE and the flower is the Daffodil. Aquamarine is said to represent the ocean or sea and is fabled to protect sailors. The Daffodil is typically the first flower to bloom in the spring after hard winters and they often poke their bulbs through the snow to give hope for an imminent thaw. A soul born from February 19th to March 20th falls under the astrological sign of Pisces, whose symbol is two fish swimming in opposite directions. Ruled by the planet Neptune, those born under Pisces are said to be both blessed and cursed. They are often empathetic, but overly trusting; artistic, but escapists; intuitive, but loners. A mutable water sign, they can have a unique ability to adapt to new environments and situations, which can cause either growth or stagnation. This adaptability is both a blessing and a curse.

Being a water sign with a planet named after the Roman sea god, a Pisces, like a calm sea or raging ocean, feels all the feelings. Sometimes called a chameleon, a Pisces is generally thought to be the last of the twelve zodiac signs, thus an amalgamation of traits derived from the previous eleven signs. According to the Chinese zodiac, those born in 1975 are born in the year of the Rabbit. A symbol of pureness and auspiciousness, people born a Rabbit are generally seen as gentle, approachable, elegant, and decent. I'll take that.

In 1975, March 7th falls on a Friday. Oliva Newton John's song *Have You Never Been Mellow* sits at #1 on the Billboard charts. Russian philosopher Mikhail Bakhtin and French actress Francine Larrimore pass away at seventy-nine and seventy-six, respectively. Gerald Ford is President of the United States and the TV show *All in the Family* is enjoying a 33.5 Nielsen rating.

The high in Tucson, Arizona, is seventy-seven degrees with a low of forty-six. They didn't know it when they went to bed the night before, but a California cheerlead-er-turned-flight attendant-turned football coach's wife and a college football assistant coach were about to become parents for the first time.

Enter five-pound, ten-ounce me.

THREE

BUT LET'S BACK UP. PICTURE IT: BARBERTON, OHIO. The 1950s. John is the third oldest of six siblings and the oldest boy. Smart and handsome with a buzz cut, he is a multi-athlete, lettering in football and basketball in high school. He dreams of coaching football and marrying a California girl who, in his midwestern mindset, are goddesses. John earns an academic scholarship to Wake Forest University from 1961-1964, where he plays quarterback for the Demon Deacons. While obtaining a Master's degree in Education from Miami of Ohio University in 1965, he serves as a graduate assistant on the football team, landing his first coaching job in 1969.

Arlene and John meet in the spring of 1969 at San Jose State University. She is an undergrad and cheerleader; he is a newly-hired assistant football coach. I've seen pictures of my mother during her college years and I can attest that she was a goddess. Still is. With long, platinum, sun-bleached blonde hair and a megawatt smile, she is the kind of "California girl" the Beach Boys sing about.

Majoring in Recreational Therapy and a member of Gamma Phi Beta sorority, this blonde bombshell is intrigued by this reserved, gentlemanly outsider. Married in December of 1971 after a year of dating, John takes a job as an assistant football coach and they move to West Point in New York. A year later, they move to Tucson, Arizona, where John takes a job as an assistant coach for the University of Arizona football team. They borrow $1,500 from Arlene's parents for a down payment on a house, decorate, and adopt a white cock-a-poo puppy named Dusty to gauge their temperament on having kids. Luckily for my brother and me, the experiment was a success. They enjoyed a few years of relative normalcy before I entered the picture in March of 1975.

On the evening of March 6th, 1975, my mother makes a meal of rice, shish kabobs, and cupcakes. She remembers this because, as she says, "I threw everything up." Around midnight, she wakes up with labor pains and goes into the nursery/guest room to start timing her contractions. Just as the sun is starting to light the sky around five o'clock in the morning, she wakes up my dad when her contractions are about five minutes apart. I have never seen my father panic, ever, so it was no surprise to me that when I asked how Dad had reacted, she deadpanned, "He took a shower and shined his shoes." Yep. That sounds exactly on brand for Dad.

They are settled into a room at Tucson Medical Center and told that delivery is hours away, so Dad heads to spring football practice (other coaching families may relate) only to be almost immediately called back to the hospital.

Dr. Herbert Pollock delivers me at 2:11 PM and I score a 7.5 on the APGAR test, which is within normal range. A couple days later, we all return home as a new family of three plus one puppy. Dad goes back to work and Dusty takes an instant liking to me. She sleeps in my crib and licks my face clean of food. Life ebbs and flows with a gentle aplomb.

But the universe always has a sense of humor, and sometimes a very wicked one.

✳

My one-month wellness check changes everything. Mom had noticed that my lips became a bit dusky when I nursed and says so to the doctor. An EKG (electrocardiogram: a quick test that measures structures and functions of the heart) shows trouble, and my mother is told to admit me to the hospital right away for more tests. She first drives straight to spring practice at the University of Arizona. She walks across the field during the middle of practice, cradling me in her arms, to break the news to my dad. This is a moment I have often thought about. You have just birthed your first child a month ago and have not even adjusted to parenthood before getting thrown a huge curveball. How do you find the grit to take those steps forward?

When I ask Dad about this decades later, wanting to know what he thought or what he said, his answer becomes the first time I have really heard his experience of that day.

"There wasn't much to say," he says, "your mother was crying." My mom explains to Dad that the doctors found a heart murmur, and though they didn't exactly know what that meant yet, Dad could sense from what she said that it was "something serious."

Diagnosis: complete AV (Atrioventricular) canal defect, or in other words, I have a hole in the center of my heart. Each of my four chambers, which are meant to separate and direct blood flow, is missing a piece. This means that blood rich with oxygen meant to be pumped to the body mixes— like oil and water—with the blood without oxygen, causing low blood-oxygen saturation levels, all of which manifests in dusky lips, fingertips, and toes. An optimal saturation level is anything above a 94%. I am in the high eighties.

Basically, my heart and lungs are working five times as hard and fast as a normal heart which, over time, will cause problems. My parents are given names of specialists and referrals to institutions such as Houston, Stanford, and the Mayo Clinic. In an act of cosmic synchronicity, my mother had met a Dr. Norman Shumway (the man responsible for the first heart transplant in the United States in 1968. More on him in a minute.) while doing her college internship in Pediatrics and Recreational Play at Stanford University Medical School. She had been responsible for preparing kids for a cardiac catheterization before Dr. Shumway performed the procedure. A catheterization is a common procedure that, in a nutshell, gives the doctors all the information about the function and health of the heart. So, when I come along with my little challenging ticker, she reaches out to him and Stanford hospital.

Now, about Dr. Shumway. He and Stanford made history by performing the first heart transplant surgery in America in January of 1968, a mere seven years before I am born. As Tracie White writes in the *Stanford Medical Newsletter* published January 4th, 2018, "The surgery that day 50 years ago captured a moment in history when the transplantation of a human heart was so hard to fathom, so bizarre, it was considered shocking, almost indecent. The heart, more than any other organ, holds a unique place in the public imagination, seen as the seat of the soul, the symbol of love and compassion."[1]

Shumway and company had been working towards transplantation since the late 1950s and announced in 1967 that they were ready to perform the first human heart transplantation. That opportunity finally came in January of 1968.

While society was debating the moral and ethical questions of this new medical frontier of organ-swapping, Dr. Shumway was simply doing what he had always done—trying to save a life. His patient, Mike Kasperak, was gravely ill and close to death. On January 5th, 1968, Kasperak suffered a major heart attack in Palo Alto. In a twist of fate, just four hours after Kasperak suffered a heart attack, forty-three-year-old Virginia Mae White suffered a brain aneurysm in a nearby El Camino hospital. The tragedy had left her brain dead, but she had been placed on a respirator after her death, which was keeping her heart alive and beating, according to White's article in the *Stanford Medical Newsletter.*[2]

Shumway and company broached the possibility of a heart transplant to Kaperak and his wife. Since this was a last-ditch effort to save his life, he and his wife were on board to try. The operation—again, the first of its kind in America—was a go.

According to White's article in the *Stanford Medical Newsletter*, as they stood over the unconscious patient, about to operate, Dr. Shumway's colleague and co-surgeon, Dr. Edward Stinton, asked him, "Do you think this is really legal?"

Shumway replied, "I guess we'll see," the article says. I cannot begin to fathom the swarm of emotions swirling around and through the doctors and nurses in that operating room.

Meanwhile, writes White, the scene outside the hospital had ballooned into a "three-ring circus," as word had gotten out that Dr. Shumway was about to attempt this ground-breaking surgery. Dan Rather, one of the most well-known and respected television journalists of the time, covered it on the national news. Indeed, the whole world was watching.

After the surgery, journalists were "scaling the hospital walls trying to snap photos of [the patient] through the windows of his hospital room," White's article said. Kasperak only lived another fifteen days, though, according to the article, Kasperak's wife counted this as a victory, saying, "That's fifteen more days he wouldn't have been here."

Dr. Stinson would later say that, in retrospect, Kasperak was "too ill at the time of surgery," White writes. She adds that Shumway and company continued their research and established "new protocols for the selection of patients and for measuring and treating rejection."[3] Indeed, getting accepted into a transplant program is an extremely thorough and rigorous process geared for garnering the best possible outcomes.

Because of Shumway's work, tens of thousands of people have gone on to receive second chances. UNOS, the United

Network for Organ Sharing, reported that hospitals around the United States performed a record-setting 3,817 heart transplants in 2021, and in the past ten years alone, 31,238 heart transplants have been performed, according to an article published on unos.org called, "Heart Transplant Sets All-Time Record in 2021."[4] Though Dr. Shumway passed away in 2006, he will be forever remembered as a life-changing pioneer.

Thank you, Dr. Shumway, from the bottom of my borrowed heart.

✳

So, it is with hope that, in 1975, my parents bring their six-month-old to be seen by this miracle-maker. Dr. Shumway's recommendation is to put a pulmonary banding around the pulmonary artery to slow the blood flow down to a more normal pace in order to preserve lung function so that a more permanent fix could be done in the future. The banding would not repair anything, but it could and would prolong other necessary surgeries until I was bigger. But a pulmonary banding still means open heart surgery in the near future on a thirteen-pound, fifteen-month-old infant with a heart the size of a walnut. My parents are crushed. They had, undoubtedly, hoped for a more permanent and less invasive fix.

My parents decide to get a second opinion and reach out to Dr. Dwight McGoon at the Mayo Clinic in Minnesota which has, for decades, been a top hospital in the United States and particularly known for their cardiac care. Dr. McGoon tells my parents, "Bring her here. I can fix her."

Dr. Dwight McGoon joined the cardiothoracic surgery team at the Mayo Clinic in Minnesota in 1957, after a tragic accident had left an open position. At the time, the thoracic surgery program at Mayo Clinic was performing two or three cardiac surgeries a month and was considered the best and "busiest in the world," according to an article by Pouya

Hemmati called, "One Hundred and Counting: Dr. Dwight C. McGoon's Enduring Legacy," published in *The Annals of Thoracic Surgery* in August 2019.[5]

McGoon's mentor at John Hopkins University, Dr. Alfred Blalcock, was instrumental in getting McGoon placed at the Mayo Clinic, believing that McGoon was his only trainee who could handle the position. Upon McGoon's beginning at the Mayo Clinic, Blalcock told him:

"This presents a great opportunity and I am sure you will make a great success of it. I envy you greatly," according to the article in *The Annals of Thoracic Surgery*.[6] At the Mayo Clinic, McGoon would prove to be a trailblazer in the field of congenital and adult cardiac surgery. In other words, another best of the best.

✳

Back to lil' old me and Dr. McGoon. Picture it: Minnesota. 1976.

He feels confident that he can repair my defect instead of putting in a temporary pulmonary banding. My parents drive from Arizona to Minnesota with fifteen-month-old me in a green Ford Taurus. During the drive that totaled more than twenty-four hours, they stop in Omaha, Nebraska, for the college World Series, in which the University of Arizona is playing. The night before I am admitted to the Mayo Clinic, we dine at a steakhouse, where I sit happily in my high-chair, munching on French fries.

Two days and many tests later, I am ready to be butterflied open. My French great-aunts on my mother's side, Marie and Pauline Bernard, go to mass and light candles at their church in San Francisco every day that I am in the hospital.

My mother remembers everything about that day, down to what she was wearing, and two particular memories stick out. She remembers Mr. Miller, my eighty-three-year-old roommate. Ernie Miller is a farmer from Minnesota who had lived with an undetected heart defect his entire life and had just undergone a successful repair. She also remembers the look on McGoon's face when he comes out of surgery. It is one of complete and utter frustration.

"I've done three thousand AV repairs," he says, "and hers was completely different."

Of course, it was. This comes to be a running joke in the family called "the Aimee Factor."

He is not able to repair the hole. So, what does he do instead? He puts a pulmonary banding around my pulmonary artery. Just like Shumway had recommended. When I ask my dad about his reaction to this, the first thing he says is, "I was angry." Not at Dr. McGoon, but at the situation. Here is his first-born, his daughter, having to undergo open heart surgery at fifteen months and likely facing further medical challenges for the rest of her life. He describes how he went to the practice range and pounded golf ball after golf ball, taking out his frustrations in his own way. My dad is not one to show an abundance of emotion, so this surprised and touched me.

The doctors tell my parents that I will probably be on the weaker side physically, and more susceptible to pneumonia and other viruses. In other words, I will probably not be a starting quarterback like my dad. They say I will be "fragile" and "limited." Luckily, none of us listened. You know what else is fragile? As Freda Kahlo says, a bomb.

Limited. My. Ass.

FOUR

ZIG ZIGLAR, THE BUSINESSMAN AND MOTIVATIONAL speaker, said, "Attitude determines altitude." I've always tried to live by this mantra and believe it to be true. There is a line between having a positive attitude and avoiding reality, to be sure. To be positive all day, every day, no matter what, is sometimes called "toxic positivity," which can lead to an avoidance of and failure to adequately deal with issues. It is hardly sustainable or realistic. But it seems to me that if you can muster a smattering of good vibes for yourself, especially in the midst of chaos, that *can* and *will* get you through some dark times. Even if you can't yet see the light at the end, just knowing the light is there can be enough to get you through the tunnel. Like Martin Luther King, Jr., said, "Faith is taking the first step, even when you can't see the whole staircase."

My parents never tell me I am different, although we all know I am. Or, to be more precise, they treat my heart condition as a simple reality, not a condition, and especially not a condition to be feared. They never tell me I shouldn't do or try certain things, but there are periodic reminders. When I am around five years old, we visit the Land of Oz theme park in North Carolina. I am obsessed with the Tin Man—specifically the large, sequined heart dangling from his neck. A picture from that day shows me in deep conversation with this Tin Man. He is crouched down, listening to me intently as I fondle the heart and explain that my own heart is "broken." I want to know where I can get a new one. I am sure the poor man had no idea what to say to me, but this Tin Man gave me someone to identify with, even if he lived in Oz. To me, he was a kindred spirit, someone who shared my fortune.

✻

Even while keeping an eagle eye out, my parents don't see limits, just their towheaded, knobby kneed, petite, feisty daughter. They never treat me as less than a perfectly healthy child nor pander to my defect, though my purple lips and fingers show otherwise. Perhaps this is where my obsession with the color purple comes from. My mother dresses me in hues that compliment my unique coloring. Worried about how I would feel looking in the mirror, she fills my wardrobe with soft blues, lilac, pinks, violet, in order to diffuse my discoloration. In fact, one of my favorite outfits ever is a purple and blue striped top and skirt set that I wear for sixth grade picture day. And decades later, my wardrobe still smacks of purple.

This is not to say that they ignore or disregard my situation. Far from it. Once I start school, Mom always makes sure to alert the school about my heart condition, as a matter of precaution. One year, I win the fifty-yard dash at my elementary school's annual track and field day. Most likely as a matter of fairness, the school lets me compete, not thinking I would strike out at breakneck speed. Ignoring a few of cries of "Stop!" and "No!" floating among the overwhelming cheers, I cross the finish line and collect my blue ribbon. When I come home with the first-place ribbon, my parents are absolutely gobsmacked. I still have the ribbon to this day.

As I grow older, the doctors and my parents adopt a plan of, "Let's keep an eye on her, but no plans for immediate surgery, maybe in a few years . . ." Basically an attitude that, "If it's not broken, don't fix it." They monitor me and toy with the idea of surgery, saying, "Well, she seems to be doing great. Let's wait on surgery for a couple years." But there are never any pressing issues that require imminent surgery. This symbiosis works for a very long time.

✳

One memory that sticks out is from fifth- or sixth-grade gym class. The PE teacher is a nice, older man, but he insists I sit out when he has the students run laps around the gym at the beginning of each class. Would I die from running? Not even close, but that sweet man has never encountered someone like me and is not going to take that chance.

Otherwise, school and life are relatively normal. I swing on the monkey bars at recess, even doing what are called "penny drops" in gymnastic terms, where you hang upside down on the bar by your knees, swing to gain momentum, then land on your feet. I play kickball, wiffle ball, and Four Square at recess. There is one small, recurring humiliation that still haunts me. Whenever I come up to "bat" in kickball, every single outfielder and baseman moves in closer, knowing that I will not kick it very far. Sigh. But hey, I never sat out a game.

I join Brownies, sell Girl Scout cookies, and go on the week-long class camping trip in sixth grade called Wildwood. We go to the woods, stay in rustic cabins in bunk beds, and do all kinds of fun camp activities. I even have a "boyfriend," Nate Wilke, from third to sixth grade. By "boyfriend," I mean that he joins our family for dinner at a restaurant on my birthday, I go over to his house a few times, and we sometimes hang out at recess. One year, he gives me an adorable May Day basket. To this day, my mom still wishes we had stayed together and married. My father is also partial to Nate. One day he asks Nate what he wants to be when he grows up.

"Surgeon," Nate exclaims.

"Great! What kind of surgeon?" my dad asks.

"Oh, just general surgery," says Nate. My father has no response. That remark endears Nate and the Wilkies to us from that moment on.

Even as a preteen with normal, preteen girl angst and growing body awareness, I'm rather blasé about the large scar running from my throat to my navel. I never bother with or worry about covering it up. I don't purposefully draw attention to it, but I consider it something of a living badge. It feels as much a part of my body as any appendage. Why would I want to deny its existence?

When I'm around eleven years old, my dad takes me swimsuit shopping in Myrtle Beach during a summer trip. I pick out a cute little bikini, probably much to my father's dismay but, God love him, he lets me get it. As my dad pays for the bikini, the proprietor of the store gives me a small 8"x10" poster with a picture of a newly hatched chick. Inside a thought bubble are the words: "I'm not a liberated chick, I'm just ahead of my time!" Indeed.

Doctors when I am in eighth grade: *Well, she seems to be doing okay. Maybe we'll think about surgery in a couple years.* Meanwhile, I ride Space Mountain, the Matterhorn, and the big waterslides, the ones with the signs proclaiming, "Anyone with heart conditions should not ride this ride." I am, at least when it comes to these signs, gleefully stubborn.

As I approach puberty, there is the distinct lack of any kind of swelling that a typical fourteen-year-old girl has which requires a trip to the mall for her first bra. My friend and neighbor, Asher, and I go to the mall for such a trip. She needs a bra and, though I don't, I buy one anyway. It is a cute, dark blue, silky one that hooks in the front; I buy it as a kind of future wish, but right now, I am as flat as an ironing board.

The reason for this specific brand of flat-chested pre-teen angst? Turner syndrome. To get science-y for a minute: Turner syndrome is a chromosomal abnormality that happens by chance during pregnancy. It occurs when "one of the X chromosomes (sex chromosomes) is missing or partially missing. It can be responsible for a slew of "medical and developmental problems, including short height, failure of the ovaries to develop, and heart defects," according to Mayo Clinic.[7]

Short height? Check. Bad ovaries? Check. Heart defect? Yep! Check.

Specifically, I have mosaic Turner syndrome, which means that some cells have an X chromosome, and some don't. Again, the Aimee Factor.

Mom and I travel ninety miles from Champaign, Illinois, to Peoria, Illinois, to see an endocrinologist specializing in Turner syndrome. At the doctor's suggestion, I start taking an injectable growth hormone. This involves daily, self-administered subcutaneous injections that will help give me some added height. I practice the injection on an orange, tricking myself that the density of an orange rind was as sensitive as skin. It's not, but it gets me used to using needles. Once a day, I take the vial of growth hormone out of the refrigerator, and use a small alcohol pad to wipe the rubber top. Then, I open a new needle, insert it through the rubber top of the syringe, tip it upside down, and draw out the correct amount. I typically choose the abdomen, as it has the fattiest tissue; I wipe down a small spot with the alcohol pad, then squeeze a bit of skin together, take a breath, and plunge the small needle in.

I also start taking pills: Estrace and Progesterone. These pills are responsible for helping me develop boobs and have a period. I hang a homemade spreadsheet inside a kitchen cabinet, checking off each injection and each pill. The growth hormone has to be kept cold, so I travel with a small, blue insulated bag with reusable, frozen chillers inside, along with enough needles and pills. I take the growth hormone for three years, which adds around five inches to my perfectly petite stature. At sixteen, I finally get my period in a rather unceremonious moment before dinner one evening.

"I got my period," I tell my mother over the phone.

"Okay, well, you know where the supplies are," she says. And that is that.

Doctors when I am in high school: *Well, she seems to be doing okay. Maybe we'll think about surgery in a couple of years.* Meanwhile, I learn how to drive. I act and sing in the school musical and join the flag corp. I attend sleepovers and basement parties, go to the mall too much (peak early nineties), make a plethora of mix tapes, and write bad poetry about crushes.

Doctors when I am a freshman in college: *Well, she seems to be doing okay. Maybe we'll think about surgery in a couple of years.* Meanwhile, I attend college halfway across the country, spend a semester in Dijon, France, pledge Kappa Alpha Theta fraternity (fun fact: KAT was the first Greek-letter fraternity for women), join the color guard for two years, date, and graduate in four years from Wake Forest University.

I rarely allow my defects to get in the way or dictate my life. I say rarely because, even with my *fuck it* attitude, I'm self-aware enough to know I do have some limits. I'm probably not going to join the volleyball or track and field teams. I have long since made peace with my lack of true athleticism, though I have, thanks to my dad's love of the game, grown up playing and enjoying golf. Even though I am never able to outdrive anyone, including my younger brother, Johnny, I develop a great swing and killer putting skills.

I'm not in denial or think I am invincible. I just refuse to let fear of what could happen scare me from living what I perceive to be a fairly normal life. But one thing I've learned: life keeps teaching you a lesson until you learn it.

FIVE

I GRADUATE FROM COLLEGE AND AM EAGER TO MOVE ON to the next stage of my life. I have dreams of moving to New York and finding work making costumes for Broadway and I don't want anything to stop me or slow me down. Doctors agree that, while I am still doing okay considering I have been living with a hole in my heart, being fully grown now makes the prospect of repair much more possible.

Since we are living in Austin, Texas, we consult with Dr. Charles Fraser at Texas Children's Hospital in Houston, Texas. Two of Dr. Fraser's three fellowships were in pediatric cardiac surgery and cardiovascular surgery respectively. He is one of the best of the best. We prepare for surgery hoping for a complete repair, but another procedure is on the table as a back-up plan.

As he explains the surgery, he also describes this back-up plan called a Fontan. It is a new procedure that is being billed as a bridge to a future heart transplant. If a Fontan is needed, he would, in plain English, "replum" my heart for the best possible blood flow. Talking about my current pulmonary banding, he illustrates on a piece of paper. It looks similar to an hourglass— imagine a six-lane highway that's cut down to two lanes for half a mile until it opens back up into six lanes. In essence, because I am now a fully-grown adult with a band intended for an infant, the blood flow is not optimal, and my lungs and body are not getting the oxygen they need. Hence, surgery.

✳

In our pre-surgery consultation, I ask Dr. Fraser how long I will be in the hospital.

"Seven to ten days," he says.

Looking him straight in the eyes I counter, "I'll give you five."

He gives me the same look my mother gives me when I have done or said something completely idiotic, a kind of *you are absolutely bonkers* look.

So, at twenty-two years old, I have open heart surgery for the second time. The time is right. In December of 1997, my parents and I travel the three hours from Austin to Houston. We arrive at the hospital extremely early in the morning for prep. For years, the doctors have said that something would have to be done "sometime." I had chosen the sometime.

I jump up onto the hospital bed, and say, "Alright, let's go!"

I am not scared. I'm not sure why, really. Perhaps because I know nothing different? This is simply the hand of life I have been dealt, so, time to play the cards.

Vitals of blood are taken and IVs are inserted. All very boring, but necessary. As the nurse is giving me the pre-op sedative through an IV, I start to find everything hilarious and am ridiculously happy to be having surgery. My laughing causes my mom and the nurse to laugh while trying to get me to lay back and close my eyes. I am told to count down from one hundred. I think I count to ninety before blackness comes.

There is one experience from surgery that remains stead-fast in my brain, through all the caverns of the conscious and unconscious. It is this: I awaken in the middle of surgery for a blink, lasting as long as a flash of lightning. I feel like I am suspended in mid-air, though I'm lying on the operating table. I see a short curtain separating my head from my body. The doctors, clad in blue scrubs with masks and head wraps, stand over and around me, working intently and hastily, but all seems calm. My mother will tell you that, to this day, I have always maintained that this happened.

As it turns out, once Dr. Fraser and team open me up, they discover that a full repair would not be possible without disrupting the heart's electrical system, which is not ideal and not worth the risk, so Fontan it is.

"Are my lips pink?" is the first thing I ask my mother after surgery. A nurse brings me a mirror to look. With the "replumbing" of my heart and somewhat corrected flow of oxygenated blood, I am expecting and hoping not to look like a Smurf anymore. I loved Smurfette; I just didn't want to look like her. And I don't anymore.

I ask to see the pulmonary banding that was removed from my heart. Laying on the metal tray, it looks like a tiny piece of bloodied scrap metal about the size of a small toe ring, something that will soon be thrown out with the biohazard waste. *Is that it?!* I think. It is extremely anti-climactic, but also mind-boggling to marvel how a small piece of man-made metal had kept doing so well for so long.

And, yes, I am released from the hospital on day five. Take that, universe!

✳

There is a marked difference in quality of living post-op. I can jog and climb flights of stairs without getting winded. Dr. Fraser had turned my malformed, four-chambered heart into a three-chambered heart, where the oxygenated and non-oxygenated blood are now, for the most part, separated. My body is now getting the oxygen-rich blood it has needed for decades. About a month after surgery, my mother and I drive to a local park to walk along the lake and feed the swans. For the first time, I run ahead of her without becoming short of breath. This, in our worlds, is absolutely remarkable.

Nine months after surgery, I move to New York City, something that would have proved more difficult before surgery, and something I had wanted to do for years. In fact, the first time I visited New York was during Spring Break of my senior year of high school. As we took the Staten Island ferry across and back, I told my parents, "I'm going to live here someday." They indulged me in a *that's nice, dear* way, but now, now I was actually going to live there.

Before surgery, tackling the subway (all those stairs!) and living in a fourth-floor walk-up would have—because of my extremely under-oxygenated blood—been extremely challenging, if not bordering on impossible. But now, it is all within the realm of the possible.

A former college roommate hooks me up with a colleague who has a room to rent, so I pack my bags and buy a ticket to my new home on East 52nd Street and quickly get a job working as a draper's assistant in a costume shop.

I do normal twenty-something-year-old things: I work, I go dancing, I stay at bars until last call, I go on dates. I go to Hoboken for watch parties with said former college room-mate. A magnificent gaggle of good college friends and I live within blocks of each other, and we live it up in the city as only twenty-somethings can. There are Halloween parties, homemade brunches, Friendsgivings, endless outings to the Village, and many hours lost to Housing Works bookstore. We even tread out to Brooklyn in a snowstorm because a bar is having a game night and we think it sounds like fun to sit in a bar and play board games. And it is. New York is a marvelous time.

Here is where I offer a short montage of the next twenty years: I move more than a few times, travel alone internationally multiple times, write and publish a few books of poetry, have many dating and break-up disasters, adopt a three-legged rescue chihuahua named Elphaba, and make a couple of career changes. I do a sixty-day Bikram yoga (hot yoga) challenge and frequently walk the hike and bike trail in Austin.

I only go to the doctor when I am sick and get checked in once a year with my pediatric cardiologist. It feels as though all of my heart issues are behind me; I make plans to further my writing career, plans for more overseas adventures, including a writing project called "50 Before 50," where I plan to try to visit fifty new places before I turn fifty.

What's that saying about making plans and God laughing?

SIX

IN JANUARY OF 2019, I TRAVEL TO THAILAND BEFORE THE start of spring semester. I feel and look fine. Perhaps I have the slightest semblance of a pooch around the midsection, but, after all, I am now over forty. I tell myself it is probably a natural consequence of aging. Otherwise, I feel more than well enough to travel halfway across the globe.

While there, my friend, Rozanne, and I decide to get reflexology massages at a swanky spa. It is a gorgeous and quaint place with complementary after-appointment tea and rice cookies. Reflexology is a traditional Chinese practice that involves massaging pressure points in the foot that are thought to correspond to certain organs and systems in the body. Led into a softly illuminated room smelling of lavender, I lie down on the mattress and close my eyes. I am enjoying the somewhat rough massage when I wince, taking both me and the masseuse by surprise. Gently, she presses and, again, I wince.

"Your heart is hurting," she murmurs, and I see a look of concern flicker across her eyes. I almost laugh out loud. Given my medical history, this absolutely tracks in my mind. I don't even give it another thought. *Of course my heart hurts,* I want to tell her, *it's been through two open-heart surgeries!*

"I know," I say, nonchalantly. She continues and does not bring it up again.

As it turns out, that would not be the only time that the universe tries to tell me something. A couple of days later, Rozanne and I decide to get a cheap, but good, street-side foot massage after dinner. I am wearing a loose-fitting, long-legged romper.

Before I even sit down, the masseuse glances at me and my midsection and asks, "Baby?" (This comment will make sense to me later.)

A bit startled, "No," I say. She is courteous and thorough, but I can tell that she isn't convinced that I'm not knocked up. Again, I chalk it up to all the fried rice, mango sticky rice, and rotis, which is an obnoxiously delicious dessert variation on the crepe. Definitely the rotis.

✳

Let's back up just a little bit. For the past year, my primary pediatric cardiologist has become concerned about my aorta, and I have had multiple CAT scans to monitor any changes. More specifically, he's concerned that I have developed an aortic aneurysm on my ascending aortic artery right at the spot where the aortic artery meets the top of the heart. The aneurysm is causing a bulge on the artery, not unlike how a balloon stretches thinner as more air is added. (I also discovered through research that women with Turner syndrome are more prone to develop aneurysms.) An unrecognized or untreated aneurysm can cause a dissection, which is a fancy word for saying that if the aneurysm gets too large, it could tear, just like a balloon could burst. What happens if the aorta tears? Well, what happens when a balloon bursts? Same thing.

At a follow-up appointment in April 2019, he gently pushes the idea of surgery in the not-too-distance future to address the aneurysm by replacing and repairing the aorta. So, I reach out to Dr. Fraser, who just happens to now be living and working in Austin, heading up the new Dell Children's Hospital. I have a consultation with him in May and book a surgery date for October 8th, 2019. Why am I waiting months? Because I really want to go on a writing retreat in France in June. This is where I insert a retroactive face palm.

Because I can be infuriatingly stubborn, in June of 2019 I travel to this writing retreat; it is on this trip I realize that all may not be as well as I think. I am starting to get out of breath from simple exertion, which is—head tilt—new? I am attending a writing residency where all meals and activities are in the Chateau. Since I am staying in a cute little house down the street, I have to walk up and down a slight incline. This would normally not be an issue for me, and isn't an issue for the others, but I find myself having to pause for a beat halfway up to catch my breath. I make a mental note, but being stubborn and hardheaded, don't think too long or hard about it. One thing I've learned about life is this: it teaches you lessons until you learn them. Still, I take walks during the trip and the three weeks go off without major incident.

❈

By July, things have progressed to where I'm feeling exceedingly lethargic and hardly leaving my apartment. I decide to drag myself to my friend Erica's yoga class, thinking it might help get me out of whatever slump I am in. I have been a regular yogi for years, and typically go three or four times a week, but I have not gone as much during the past eight months.

Five minutes in, I have to lie down. I stay there for the rest of the class, and I am absolutely pissed.

What the fuck is going on?! I fume in my head. *This shouldn't be happening.*

It is dawning on me that there may be something serious going on. I have been riding a wave of relatively good health for decades and, though I don't know it quite yet, I am about to wipe out big time.

Mid-July I have an episode that lands me in the hospital for a few days. It starts like this: I text my friend, Janiece, that I am going to take an Uber to urgent care and I ask her to join me. Once we are settled into an exam room a short while later, the nurse takes my vitals and is silent and quickly exits. My heart rate is through the roof and my blood oxygen saturation is in the mid-80s.

A moment later, a doctor opens the door and without even coming in or taking her hand off the handle says, "I've called an ambulance."

Oh, crap.

I turn to Janiece and give her my house keys.

"I need you to do me a huge favor and go grab a few things and get Elphie," I say. Like the bestie she is, she takes my keys, my list of things to get, and says she'll meet me at the hospital soon.

I call my pediatric cardiologist and alert him to what's going on and he meets me at the hospital. They give me some IV meds to help my heart rate come down and soon I start to feel relatively better and am released after a couple of days.

For the rest of July and August, I am pretty much home-bound. It is becoming a chore to go up and down the steps to walk my tiny, seven-pound Chihuahua, Elphie. I have little appetite and survive on yogurts and fruits; I drink a sailor's worth of Gatorade. I am still counting on having surgery on October 8th, figuring that replacing and repairing my aorta will fix things.

In early September, my mom comes to visit, so I trudge over to my brother's house for a dinner. She notices and comments on my belly, which has slowly become distended to the point where I look pregnant, though my pants still fit. On September 14th, she accompanies me to my final cardiac catheterization before surgery, and we sneak in an "off the books," super-early morning appointment with Dr. Fraser to talk about the upcoming scheduled surgery. As I dress for the appointment, I have to pry my feet into my normally easy and comfortable Toms.

Huh, that's weird, I think, seeing the top of my foot bulging slightly out of my shoes. I don't know it yet, but will find out very soon that this is directly related to my heart and liver failure.

Mom returns to California a few days later and we start to make preparations for her to return in early October for my surgery. Unbeknownst to me at the time, Mom writes a two-page email to my dad, brother, and sister-in-law. I want to relay a part of it as evidence of that adage about hindsight being 20/20:

Last night Amy Lang Johnson (a best friend since 3rd grade) *from KC sent me messages, as she and Aimee have had a talk. Amy said Aimee told her she is mad and scared and thought the surgery she had 22 years ago would have been the last. Amy said she knows Aimee is depressed as well, but was her usual stoic self and Aimee kind of challenged her on that. Aimee and I had exchanged multiple small texts about Wake [Forest football] game and when I asked if she would be me a favor she responded "if I can." I simply asked her to take the medicine that she had, in fact, asked for weeks ago that is to aid sleep but also a mild antidepressant every day for a few weeks. I acknowledged that she wouldn't be human if she wasn't sad, unhappy, and scared. I got crickets back. Nothing.*

✳

Sometimes, you don't even know you're depressed until someone tells you. Only those on the outside can tell. During this time, I am not feeling myself but, as is obvious looking back, not doing enough to acknowledge or deal with it. I had been having trouble sleeping and had recently asked for some medication, as Mom mentions in the letter. I can only attribute it to my stubbornness that, after taking the medication for a few days and not seeing an improvement, had stopped. As an English professor, I teach students to analyze literary characters' speech and actions and determine a primary character trait, one that often impacts and spurs on the action of the story. If you can't tell, dear reader, my primary character trait is stubbornness. From the same letter:

So, I started thinking about all the things that are over-whelming her right now. Daily chores and just stuff she is not doing or capable of doing at the moment. Most everything we take for granted when caring for ourselves. Adding depression to simple tasks makes life a vicious circle. Grocery shopping, picking up the mail, doing laundry, having car serviced, cleaning, taking medication, fixing meals, daily hygiene, classwork and the learning lab (one of my three jobs), *wanting to do yoga . . . then add to that her frustration of her body image and belly distension and top it off with a more than major heart surgery on the horizon. She needs help.*

Yes. Yes, I do. I have started asking for small acts from local friends. I ask Janiece to pick up some more meds and bring me Gatorades. Johnny and Tiffany come over. They vacuum, take some things to Goodwill and to sell, and take a few brown bags' worth of stuff down to the recycle dumpster. Johnny arranges for a washer and dryer to be installed. I ask Rozanne to come and help me clean the kitchen and small mountain of dishes. Mom is right that I am frustrated. I am frustrated that my body is failing me, though I am still thinking that upcoming surgery will "fix" it.

On September 25th, I have what I think is going to be a final pre-surgery consultation with Dr. Fraser. My brother picks me up and accompanies me to the appointment so that he can ostensibly be another pair of ears and eyes. Really, he is there because I don't trust myself to drive anymore and neither does my family.

As soon as Dr. Fraser walks in the exam room, I instinctively know that whatever he is going to say is not good news.

His face is completely serious, even sad, and he is subdued. He says hello, then asks my brother to get my mother on the phone.

Oh shit, I think, *this is not good.*

"I can't do your surgery anymore, Aimee," he says, "you're too sick and your case is too complicated for us now."

Have you ever had a moment where your life changes on a dime? It is like that. I start to feel slightly lightheaded. The gravity of the situation is now slamming into me with the force of a bulldozer.

And here's the kicker. He then says, "And I would like to admit you to the hospital today."

Now, if I am going to listen to anyone when it comes to my heart, it's Dr. Fraser. I don't remember much else about that visit, only that he draws some things on the board explaining what's going on. After you're told you have to be admitted to the hospital ASAP, everything kind of goes murky. Luckily, my brother and mother (on the phone) are engaged enough to keep listening. He starts throwing out other major medical institutions such as Mayo Clinic in Minnesota and Cleveland Heart Clinic in Ohio. You know, places that take on the most complicated and dire cases. Dr. Fraser arranges for my admission that day. Mom books another flight to Austin.

Ladies and Gentlemen, as they say at the Indy 500, *start your engines.*

SEVEN

MY BROTHER AND I HIGHTAIL IT BACK TO MY APARTMENT so I can pick up some things. He helps me up the one flight of stairs. Quickly I throw the immediate necessities into my more than twenty-year-old, monogramed L.L. Bean backpack. Jammies, computer, brush, toothpaste, book, etc. My brother takes the garbage out and takes Elphaba to go potty. I don't know it at the moment, but this is the last time I will ever be in that apartment. My brother and I hurry back to the hospital during a hot Texas rush hour. He drops me off, then goes back to my apartment to pick up Elphaba. It goes without saying, bless him, that he and his family will take care of her.

✳

Dell's Children's Hospital is a brand-new, wonderful, world-class facility. I am settled in a large room with a private bathroom and flat screen TV. I am hooked up to oxygen and an IV. The nurse draws about a million vials of blood and does another EKG.

A couple days later, Dr. Fraser's brow knots up while he's looking over my results. He gently launches the word "transplant" into the air, like a silent bomb I'm supposed to catch.

Transplant. Like having a new engine put in a car; it's the same car, just new parts. Though the word was in the family lexicon ever since I had had surgery at age twenty-two, I never really thought it a distinct, probable possibility. Though this was discussed during the consultations before my surgery in 1997 that Fontan was a new procedure that is meant to be a bridge to an eventual transplant, I have obviously decided to forget this part. Perhaps it is part of my coping mechanisms that I honestly and truly have no recollection (blocked out?) of any conversation that involved the word "transplant" at that time.

After twenty-two years of living with a Fontan, I have become sick enough and my situation complex enough that my only option is a heart transplant. And soon. There is also concern that my liver is not in good shape. The extra weight I am experiencing is due to fluid retention as a result of liver failure, which we learn is a long-term effect of the Fontan.

There is more bloodwork along with ultrasounds. Doctors also do a procedure called a paracentesis which, in layman's terms, is an abdominal tap. It's very much like an amniocentesis. A needle in the belly. I watch my stomach slowly deflate like a beachball running out of air while they drain three liters of yellow, infected fluid from my midsection.

Saturday, September 28, Mom arrives again. Unbeknownst to me, my primary cardiologist has been in contact with her and has arranged to meet her at my hospital room when she arrives. Around seven o'clock in the evening, he comes in with a not-all-too-cheery smile on his face. Sitting in a chair at the end of the bed, he is short on small talk and gets right to the point. Honestly, I do not remember the exact words he said, but the gist of it is that, due to a blood test result, he thinks there is a possibility I might have ovarian cancer.

"How do you feel?" he offers.

Time slams to a halt. I am suspended in space where nothing else is happening and nothing exists outside of my hospital room. Any air in my lungs is sucked out of my body through that vortex activated by shock.

"I feel blindsided," I finally say, numb.

I am too shocked to cry, but my mind is reeling. I question that the benevolent universe I believe in would really saddle me with a transplant, a failing liver, *and* cancer. *I don't have cancer*, I think, *this can't be true.*

Ah, but that's the thing—cancer would be bad enough, but having any kind of active cancer would automatically disqualify me from being accepted for a transplant.

After my cardiologist leaves, my mom turns to me like someone who has just been to a funeral and says, "If there is anything in there, I want it taken out."

A couple of days and some more blood tests later, it is confirmed that I do not have cancer. My mother is still sour over that whole experience. Why add to the current stress of a transplant a non-confirmed, possibly tragic diagnosis which, thank goodness, turns out not to be the case?

So, I don't have cancer. Yay. But, I still need a heart and liver transplant. Boo.

While Dr. Fraser and the new Dell Children's Hospital are superb, they are not yet prepared to do transplants, especially the special twofer heart and liver transplant that I need, because *my body always gotta be extra.* The Aimee Factor.

Dr. Fraser makes calls to the Mayo Clinic, Cleveland, and Stanford. He connects with a colleague, Dr. George Lui, a pediatric congenital cardiologist at Stanford who tells him, "Get her out here as soon as possible."

Dr. Lui is confident their transplant team is the best option for a heart and liver transplant. And Mom lives three hours from Stanford, which the hospital would look favorably upon if they accepted me for a transplant, since patients are required to have a full-time caregiver and have frequent appointments for at least a year afterwards. We immediately begin the process of getting me transferred out to Stanford, which involves a flurry of tests, telephone calls, and paperwork.

My friend Erica asks me how I feel about getting a transplant.

"Well, I don't really have a choice," I laugh.

To my family's chagrin, my attitude about facing tough situations is quite often, "Do not worry about it until absolutely necessary," and, when it comes to my heart and health, "Do not panic until the doctor says it is time to panic." Though the doctors have hit the panic button, I am still not panicking. Yet. One, because I trust and know that Dr. Fraser and his team are doing absolutely everything they can. Two, I have utter faith in Stanford and Dr. Lui. And three, panicking has never accomplished a dang thing.

That week, my mother stays at her friend's house in Austin while she and my sister-in-law basically take charge of logistical tasks that I am unable to do. They pack up my apartment, sell off some furniture, and put the rest in storage. It dawns on me that, not only will I not be returning to that apartment, it looks as though I will be moving to California for the foreseeable future.

Some dear friends visit me in the hospital: an old roommate, Rozanne; my bestie, Janiece; and my friend Erica, who brings my favorite popcorn and a small stuffed unicorn. Erica obsesses over my oxygen level, which is hovering around eighty-five with a low flow of oxygen. She watches it like a hawk, her eyes darting back and forth between the monitor and my small phone as I make her watch Dr. Pimple Popper videos with me. A family friend, Heather, makes a delicious, Prince-inspired cake to share with the nurses.

The days are spent tying up whatever loose ends I can and teaching my one English Composition course online for Keiser University, where I have been employed as an online professor of English for ten years. I feel vaguely pissed that I allow myself to think it's okay to be working from the hospital, but it's a nice distraction.

I also write to the head of the department of English at Austin Community College, where I have been adjuncting in the English department and working as a tutor for more than four years. I outline the situation as best I can and tell them I will keep them posted. To their credits, Keiser and ACC are supremely sympathetic and genuine in their concern for me.

I cancel my car insurance and cable. My brother writes a letter to get me out of my lease. While I certainly don't feel like running a marathon, I am feeling much better after the paracentesis and am generally in good spirits. I've never been afraid of surgery before, so I tell myself I have no reason to be afraid of a double transplant. Ha.

As part of the process to get listed, I have to have a will and Medical Directive Power of Attorney on file. Although making a will for me is simple (Johnny gets Elphaba. Mom gets everything else to distribute.), the reason as to why I'm having to arrange a will buzzes around me like a pesky gnat.

Death.

I'm doing this so they know what to do if I die. And the Medical Power of Attorney? That is in case things go smashingly wrong and my mother can make medical decisions on my behalf if I am not able to either do so, physically or medically. Since I have always operated with a "leap first, look later" attitude (sorry, fam), I am not used to the heft that these documents represent, nor am I used to preparing for future worst-case scenarios.

I text Janiece, asking her to help me draft the will and ask if she knows a notary who can come to the hospital (because she knows everyone), and, of course, she does. Bless them both to eternity and back for coming to the rescue.

Another thing that happens this week is that Erica sets up a private Facebook group as a space for me and/or Mom to post updates. Besides family and a few local friends, no one else knows what is really going on yet, so it feels important to have a central spot to communicate with everyone in real time. She names the group "Team Glitter Unicorn," after an inside joke, but I love it.

Mythical and powerful, the unicorn has been represented in art and history countless times over the past 1,000 years, the first description appearing in Greek literature in 400 BC by the Greek historian Ctesias, who describes the creature as "the size of a horse, with a white body, purple head, and blue eyes, and on its forehead was a cubit-long (18 inches) horn colored red at the pointed tip, black in the middle, and white at the base," according to *Encyclopedia Britannica.*[8] I mean, why wouldn't I want to be a horse with a purple head that can stab things?!

A half-dozen days of paperwork later, transport is scheduled for October 9th, one day after the surgery date that was not to be. My brother, sister-in-law, and their four kids sneak (with permission) my dog into the hospital to see me one last time. I hold my dog and hug my nephew and nieces as much as they let me. They ask about the oxygen tank and are a little puzzled at seeing me in a wheelchair. I didn't know it at the time, but that day would be the last time I held or saw my dog in person. Life, huh?

EIGHT

MOM FLIES ON OCTOBER 7TH SO SHE CAN MEET ME AT Stanford hospital. The morning of October 9th, my brother comes to the hospital to see me off and helps carry my bags out to the ambulance. He then follows us out to the small airport. Turns out, if you're really sick, you can get insurance to cover a private transport by plane from Texas to California. Two pilots, two nurses, and myself, all crammed into a tiny jet. It's a medical transport jet, so it is far from swanky. The nurse offers me drinks and snacks. Four hours later, I land in California, blithely optimistic.

Compared to the newly-built, beautiful Dell's Children's Center in Austin, the original Stanford hospital was built in 1950. It is noisy, run down, and painfully plain. And not private, as I soon find out. I am first taken to the emergency room for intake, then moved to a large room with three other patients. The nurse on duty, Cody, hands me a hospital gown.

"No, thanks," I say, "I'll stay in my pajamas."

He looks only slightly miffed, bless him.

He shrugs, "Okay. That's fine."

My reality was starting to feel like a full-on 3D IMAX movie in Dolby Surround sound. Intense and inescapable.

I am living in a hospital, and probably will be for a while. Things are serious and the clock is ticking.

Within the hour, we meet the transplant coordinator, Pam. An angel on earth, she is in charge of onboarding patients and, when it comes time, fielding organ offers from hospitals. She is the first step in this new, very unfamiliar process. She comes armed with a four-inch binder and talks with us for more than an hour. She has a great laugh and instantly makes me feel grateful that she is in charge of navigating this complex and daunting medical maze of tests, psychological evaluations, lifestyle questionnaires, and doctors' letters.

So, in a nutshell, the transplant process goes like this: once you are accepted for transplant, you are listed with the United Network for Organ Sharing (UNOS), the national non-profit organization that organizes and manages the organ-sharing system in the United States. The United States is divided by UNOS into eleven different regions. Since I am in California, I will only be able to receive organs that come from a donor in California, Nevada, Idaho, Arizona, or New Mexico. This is simply because, since there is a limited time in which to transplant a new organ, there are limitations on how far away it can come from.

Once you are accepted, you are given a status based on a number of variables, including blood type, genetic compatibility, time spent waiting, and how sick you are. There are six status ratings:

Status 1-3: In the hospital, often in ICU, most severe cases.

Status 4: Typically at home, may need IV or LVAD (heart pump).

Status 6: Patients stable enough to wait at home.

I am listed as a Status 4 and given a choice of waiting at my mom's home or in the hospital. Although I am tempted to wait at mom's house, a patient is moved up in status if they are in the hospital, so Mom and I decide that I will remain in the hospital, which, as you will read, turns out to be a blessing in disguise and the decision almost a moot point.

Once a patient is put on the list, they wait for an offer from UNOS. When a designated donor passes away, their information is shared with UNOS, which then produces a ranked list of possible recipients. UNOS then starts at the top of the list and calls the affiliated hospital with the offer of an organ. If the doctors think it is a potential good match, the surgeon gets in a helicopter to go inspect the organ in person. (At Stanford, you can hear this life-changing helicopter taking off and landing. It is truly a trip.) Once the doctor determines that the organ is a good match, they alert the hospital, and the patient and O.R. are prepped for surgery.

Wondering how patients are matched with organs? An array of variables are taken into account when matching an organ with a recipient: blood type, health of recipient (the more severe the patient, the higher they are on the list), geography, patient waiting time, and, for certain organs, organ size. Finding the right organ feels like a bit of conjured magic.

The next day, as they are coordinating transport to a regular room, I implore them to please not move me between 4:00 PM and 5:00 PM, as that is when I am supposed to lead my online class. At 4:07, of course, transport comes. One of the nurses on duty, Emmett, apologizes, saying, "Okay, Aimee, I'm so sorry, but we gotta go."

He proceeds to wheel me through the hospital to my new room as I stay online (thank you, Stanford Wi-Fi) and logged into Blackboard Ultra, the educational portal's version of Zoom. Emmett is floored by this, telling random people as we pass, "She's teaching class right now! She's a rock star!"

※

A heart catheterization and liver biopsy are scheduled back-to-back for October 14th. A heart catheterization is where they insert a tiny camera through a vein, typically in the groin, and move it up to the heart. Then, a contrast dye is injected and pictures are taken. Basically, it gives the doctors extremely pertinent and accurate information about current heart function. A biopsy is taking a small sample of something to test it for various things.

The liver biopsy goes smoothly; under light sedation, it's like a three-martini lunch. The cardiac catheterization, not so much. It begins normally, though the sedation from the liver biopsy has begun to wear off. I try to get the attention of the doctor, but he is concentrating. Though it feels like half an hour, I'm sure it is only a few minutes before I become increasingly anxious, which is not my typical vibe. My blood pressure spikes violently; I turn my head to the right and immediately vomit a very large amount of blood. The doctor jerks his hands back as a couple of nurses jump in to help me. Luckily, the doctor has just completed the cath, so I am cleaned up and sent to the ICU, not back to my room, for observation.

Meanwhile, Mom returns to my room after getting some food to find my belongings gone. Unbeknownst to her, nurses have packed my things when I was sent to the ICU, which is on another floor altogether. This sends Mom in a tailspin of panic. Remember that hospital scene in the movie *Terms of Endearment* when Shirley MacLaine yells at a nurse until the nurse gives Debra Winger, who plays MacLaine's daughter, pain medication? I wasn't there, but I imagine it probably went about like that. The nurses on the floor direct Mom down to the ICU and, after an overnight stay, I am released and moved back into a regular room.

The new room is small and not private. There is a small bathroom (toilet and sink only) and enough room for two hospital beds, plus equipment and four chairs. There is a slider curtain to "separate" the space and a small TV mounted on the wall opposite each bed. There is barely room for a chair at the end of the bed for my mom to sit in. Like the champion she is, she stays with me at the hospital every day. We are blessed to have family that lives twenty minutes from Stanford in Los Altos, so Mom moves into a spare room.

The bed is not as comfortable as my old bed at home, and it's sometimes hard to sleep at night. Right outside the room is an annoyingly loud pill dispensing machine that is used 24/7. I soon ask for something to help me sleep, which doesn't particularly help. The nurses come in to do vitals assessments throughout the night, which are all a part of the charm of a hospital stay. Not. I admit to not being the best patient when, in a fit of frustration one day, I write on the patient whiteboard: "*Please do NOT wake me up unless we are on FIRE* ☺," with **FIRE** underlined for emphasis. There are, at the time, wildfires ravaging California.

The days are sprinkled with blood draws, doctors' rounds, and other medical maintenance, but are, otherwise, fairly boring. Mom and I take several short walks a day with my oxygen tank in tow. I am told to try and do as much walking and eating as I can before surgery. I am sick, but stable enough. A throng of wonderful doctors come in and out as they go through rotations. There's Dr. Fowler, a lovely older English gent, who is mostly bored with me, because my condition doesn't really change from day to day. He comes in, looks things over, asks his students a question or two, tells a joke, and says, "Well, I got nothing." Meaning I am, at the moment, relatively medically stable.

There is Dr. Vagelos, who always comes in while I am grading papers (because I am still working and, yes, I know it's ridiculous) and asks me if I had found any plagiarists.

"Not today," I joke. He is wonderful, but honest and real. There are a number of doctors and nurses that my family and I will never forget, and Dr. Vagelos is one of them.

The "roommate roulette" proves to be quite comical. There is the lady who has just had a baby, which the nurses bring in several times a night for nursing. Though I am slightly annoyed at being awakened throughout the night, to see how surrounded she is by family (there must have been about ten people crammed around her double bed) gives me reason to smile. I want to ask to hold the baby, but decide against it.

There is Mrs. Singh, from Davis, California, who had just had a heart transplant a year ago and is having some mild rejection. She and her husband are so sweet and it is wonderful to meet and talk face-to-face with someone who has been through the process. She is discharged after a few days and the rotation continues.

There's the lady in her late fifties or sixties, perhaps, whom my mom and I are convinced is on something. As soon as the nurses bring her into the room and try to get her situated, she asks for a cigarette. Seriously. Her smoker's voice booms and she is abrasive and rude to the nurses. Her clothes are dirty and disheveled; her hair is wild and unkempt. She also has with her at least a half-dozen plastic bags filled with who knows what.

At one point, my mom asks her to please lower her voice, to which she proceeds to yell at my mom. It goes a little something like this:

Mom: "Do you mind lowering your voice a little? My daughter is very sick and waiting for a heart transplant—"

Lady (interrupting loudly): "Oh yeah?! Well, I had a transplant and I have cancer!"

Sure, and I am Lady Gaga. She is clearly lying.

Mom and I shrug, do our best to ignore her, and keep the dividing curtain drawn 24/7. Sometime the next day, we hear her talking on the phone to whom we think, from what she says, is her son-in-law. At one point, she says crassly and with glee, "Ah, just lift up her skirt and do her!"

Mom and I look at each other silently, wide-eyed, and attempt to peel our jaws off the floor.

As I am eating breakfast the next morning, I blow my nose. I hear her grumbling nearby, saying something about being loud.

"Are you talking to me?" I venture, surprised.

"Yes, bitch, I'm talking to you!"

I tell her to please be quiet and just eat her breakfast. Like a lit match, she starts going off, calling me a "silver-spoon bitch whose mother wipes her ass for her." She also says that I probably had my children taken away from me for being a "shitty mother" and other vile things. Lady, I don't even have kids!

I'm really sorry, dear reader, but it is at this point I snap and yell, "Shut the fuck up!" loud enough that I know someone will hear it. Sure enough, two nurses come running. It turns out they have been keeping a record of the patient's verbal abuses to the nurses, as well as to my mom and me. She is removed within the hour. Fun times.

Besides the scary catheterization incident and that bit of roommate drama, the rest of October drifts by with relative ease. I watch football on the weekends. My dad visits and hangs a Wake Forest flag on the curtain that divides the room. A family friend hooks me up with Stanford swag. I keep "teaching" my online class. My rationale is that, as long as I'm able to, why not? My Aunt Joanie visits. As do my cousin Kirsten and Uncle Les. My cousin Heather, my Aunt Lynn, and Uncle Larry live close enough to visit as well. We sit outside surrounded by other patients in wheelchairs with IV poles. Kirsten brings me Chipotle. Aunt Joanie brings homemade cookies. Mom's significant other, Ralph, is here.

The hospital food, in all honesty, is good. I order the creamy and delicious shrimp with ravioli many times. Their short ribs are excellent. I've never been a huge eater. I eat to live, not live to eat, but Dr. Vagelos continues to urge me to eat as much as I can and exercise as much as I can in preparation for surgery. Basically, the fatter and more "in shape" I am for surgery, the better. There are also countless blood draws, which are taken through the IV, so at least I'm not getting stuck with a needle every day, and a couple of additional abdominal taps to take more off additional infected fluid that keeps accumulating in my midsection.

A bright spot is the therapy dogs that come by two to three days a week. There is Levi, a beautiful black and white Australian Shepherd, docile as a lamb. There is the spunky Jessie, a cute little, wiry Border Terrier who reminds me of the famous Benji from the eighties. But Gertie is my favorite. A stocky little French Bulldog, she snuggles up next to me in bed and coolly ignores her handler when it is time to go. Truly, I would have let Gertie lay there forever.

A new Stanford hospital has been built right next door (the current one is going to be renovated) and is set to open on November 17th. Squeaky clean with private rooms, I can hardly wait. As moving day approaches, the hallway slowly becomes nearly empty as they move equipment and supplies over. The night before the move, a nurse delivers two brown bags to gather up my stuff. I've now been here a month, so I actually have to pack up. Clothes (I am not yet ready to wear a hospital gown until they tell me I absolutely have to), computer, brushes, books, etc. Someone also comes by with some Stanford hospital swag—a blanket, a water bottle, and a nice tote. The morning of the move, I am prepped and ready. They start early and I am honestly impressed with their planning and execution.

Around noon, they come for me and I am rolled in my hospital bed down the hall, through an atrium, and to an elevator. There are photographers documenting the occasion and a rainbow of balloons greet us as we enter the new hospital. It is a decidedly celebratory vibe. For a hospital. J7 is my new wing (J) and level (7). Level 7 is for those who are stable and/or on their way out of the hospital. In other words, not intensive care.

I am rolled into a huge, beautiful corner room with huge windows on two sides which look out over the Stanford campus and is possibly one of the most expensive views in Palo Alto. There is also a full bathroom and a giant TV from which I can order room service. It is the nicest hospital room ever.

It is so nice that I immediately take a video while walking around and post it with commentary. An hour later, my mom and Ralph are able to come in, and my mom's jaw drops. We later learn that Sarah, the nurse who had thrown out the nasty roommate, had put in a word for me to get the nice corner room. God bless nurses forever and ever and ever, amen.

NINE

ALL I HAD TO DO WAS SIT ON MY BUTT IN THE SWANKIEST hospital room on earth and wait for a heart and liver. But no, my body had to make things interesting. About five days after moving in, I order a wrap for lunch. Coincidentally, there is, at the moment, an ongoing recall of tainted lettuce. Do you see where I am going with this?

Within two hours of eating what I am convinced is bad lettuce in my wrap, I am violently throwing up and spike a fever. Besides a nasty infection, I am diagnosed with E. coli. Because *my body always gotta be extra*. To the dismay of myself, my family, and the sweet coordinator, Pam, I am temporarily taken off the transplant list, as they won't transplant someone with raging infections. Makes sense. Dammit.

Vials and vials of blood are drawn. Blood cultures are taken, which is a whole other process where blood is drawn using a new needle (not the IVs) from each arm at the inner elbow crease and collected in what looks like mini-bar liquor bottles; the blood whooshes in, filling them up like a thin, bright Tabasco sauce.

This is the worst I have felt since this whole medical merry-go-round started last summer. I am moved from that room to the ICU. I'm so sick that I barely mourn the loss of the room bigger than my first apartment in New York City in 1999. Goodbye, beautiful room with remote-control window shades. Goodbye, fifty-five-inch TV screen with Netflix. Goodbye, beautiful view.

✳

Over the following week, doctors try a variety of antibiotics with minimal success. It is not enough to get me back on the list. Every specialist is thrown at me: gastro, liver, heart, infectious diseases. At one point, Dr. George Lui, the head of the adult congenital heart program at Stanford and the one responsible for getting me into Stanford, is talking to Mom and Ralph at my bedside.

"We need to get the infection under control as soon as possible," he says, quietly.

I look up at him, squeaking out, "Or what?"

He does not answer, but I know what the answer is. I can see it in his gentle, dark eyes. I am running out of time.

✳

It is Dr. Ho, the infectious disease expert, a warm and funny Asian lady with a petite frame and short dark hair, who finally gets to the bottom of my infection.

"Always with the football," she would say good-naturedly whenever she came into the room and a football game was on the TV, because it is fall and we're a recovering coaching family.

"In my twenty years here, I have known about it, but I have never seen this infection in a patient!" she marvels. Because, of course. The Aimee Factor. The culprit is Eggarthella lenta, a nasty bacterium that, in my case, has weaseled its way into my bloodstream.

From then on, she has all blood draw results sent to her desk personally, in addition to all the other doctors. I am put on new antibiotics and finally recover enough to get back on the transplant list. This is how November goes. A series of disappointing backslides and subsequent miracles with a sprinkle of tenacious reality.

The day before Thanksgiving, the team puts in an Impella pump, otherwise known as an artificial heart pump, in order to keep my failing heart functioning until transplant. The situation has gotten that dire, that fast.

By the next day, Thanksgiving, they determine the pump is not doing enough and I am now in severe congestive heart failure. My heart is in atrial fibrillation—or in layman's terms—I have a wonky heart rhythm. To try and correct the rhythm, doctors try a cardio-conversion. Have you ever seen a medical drama on TV where the doctor takes two paddles and puts them to the chest of person flatlining on the gurney and yells *Clear!* and the dying person is shocked and everyone stays silent, listening for the heartbeat? It is like that, except I am, thankfully, sedated. They are trying to get my heart rhythm under control.

I don't remember a lot, but from my mom, I've gathered that the scene looked something like this: Dr. Hill and others surround my bed, buzzing around me like bees frantically trying to get my heart rhythm under control. Out in the hall, Dr. Vagelos and Dr. Lui watch through the window, but they are not looking at me. Their eyes are glued to the monitor. The cardio-conversion is not working. Dr. Vagelos—who is sicker than a dog with the flu or something—stays outside of the room, and puts his head in his hands in frustration. He and others spend their entire Thanksgiving Day working on me.

When I come to afterwards, I ask my mom if the cardio-conversion worked, but the answer is written all over her face. Disappointment. Uncertainty. She shakes her head slightly, her lips pressed together in a thin line, like a flatline.

"No," she says, emotionless.

The doctors are quickly hitting the bottom of their bag of tricks.

✳

Since the Impella pump is not doing enough and the cardio-conversion did not work, the team throws a Hail

Mary. They take me to surgery again and put me on what is called the ECMO machine. ECMO is short for Extracorporeal Membrane Oxygenation. It is similar to a heart and lung bypass machine used during open heart surgery. This is an extreme measure and a very short-term solution only meant to be used for up to two weeks. In other words, I need a heart and liver yesterday.

Ralph, my bonus dad and Mom's partner of the past decade, takes a picture shortly before I am wheeled off to surgery. In the picture, I am lying in the hospital bed surrounded on both sides by piles of IVs and monitors and almost lost among a pile of tubes and lines. Mom hovers my laptop over me, so I can try to write some emails. I am emailing my supervisors, telling them what is going on and that I am too sick to continue teaching my classes. You think?!

Mom's post in the Team Glitter Unicorn Facebook group on November 29, 2019:

Hi all. Aimee will not be pleased with this post as she asks that I not scare anyone, but she will learn to forgive me. Aimee's situation is quite dire. Her sweet, perfect-imperfect heart ♥ is just wearing out. She has a dangerous infection in the belly lining that must be controlled before transplant and her perfect-imperfect heart can't pump enough to get it there.

She is presently in surgery, where they are putting her on an ECMO pump that will do what her perfect-imperfect heart can't and see if they can get the infection to respond.

Today, as they had a surgery group in the room to transport her, she was having me email the Department Head at ACC (Austin Community College) to let him know that she needed a substitute for the remaining two weeks of classes. Forever thinking ahead.

The surgery assistant just came out and said they successfully placed the pump and we can see her soon. The ECMO is not something that can last indefinitely. We are all in this together and however you pray, I am asking for help. She is an amazing, awesome warrior woman that we need in our world, and I want in my life♥

Love, the Mom

P.S. I failed to add how enormously grateful we are to her medical teams here at Stanford. They are going beyond what one could possibly imagine. I am indebted to them forever, and feel their love and care for her daily ♥

Just about twenty-four hours later, another update from Mom:

So, the good news is, Aimee was not upset with my post yesterday 😊👍 *and has asked me to give you all a brief update of her Saturday, now 24 hrs on the ECMO pump.*

This is a magnificent machine that is doing all the hard work her perfect-imperfect heart ♥*could no longer do. It is pumping the (her) oxygen-enriched blood from machine back into her body like a perfect heart would do. Something she has never felt or had.*

In turn is the hope that this enhanced circulation will increase the volumes for antibiotics to get to where they need to wipe out the peritonitis. That IS the elephant in the room. They took a small amount of belly fluid this afternoon to see if there are any changes. And blood work is constantly being checked.

We have just a few precious days to accomplish this feat and then be activated again and placed at the top of the donor organ need list. A ballet of sorts in which no one wants to drop their partner!

Over a period of about 2-3 hrs this morning, we had 5 different medical specialty teams in here talking and explaining everything. Met transplant surgeon and team members, Liver doctors, infectious disease fun folks, heart teams, and now ones I can't remember. The way they choreograph her care and communicate with each other is what we would like to see in many parts of our society. What Aimee has asked me to tell you is that, for today, they were collectively but very cautiously pleased. A very mini step in a long marathon, but a first step none-the-less. What is surrounding her bed are wonderful machines invented by some crazy scientists!!! But the 50" TV screen is NOT blocked and she is watching a little college football.

What Aimee really wants each and every one of you to know and feel is her love and deep gratitude for the prayers and well wishes she is receiving! You are all an important part of her life and she needs you on this journey with her. For me, she is the ultimate Rockstar and we are the groupies cheering her on

With great affection and appreciation

Aimee and her Mom

Because of the ECMO machine, I am confined to the bed in a nearly flat position. This is a special bed that tilts, so that I can "sit up," which is really like standing at a forty-five-degree angle, but it's better than nothing. I ask the nurses from time to time to raise my head just a bit and basically do little more than sleep, watch TV, and chat with Mom and doctors.

Along with the ECMO come the specially trained perfusionists: nurses who work solely and specifically with the ECMO machine. Multiple times a day, the nurse checks the machine and makes any necessary adjustments. All the perfusionists are extremely nice, young, and good looking. Mom and I joke with them that we are going to make a Perfusionist of the Month calendar. As well as being gentlemen, they are gorgeous distractions.

My brother comes during this time as a result of a conversation Mom and Ralph had with Dr. Lui the day of my ECMO surgery. It was late in the evening of the 29th, and Dr. Lui finds Ralph while Mom is in the restroom and sits down beside him.

"I know that Aimee has a brother," he says.

Ralph nods. "Yes."

"Now might be a good time," he says, "to have him and her father visit."

Mom joins them to find Ralph in tears. The statement and silence are steeped in thoughts and feelings that no one wants to say out loud. Besides the fact that the ECMO is only a very temporary solution, I am still ravaged with an infection that needs to be under control before they can even think of reactivating me on the transplant list. Then, I still have to wait for a donor.

I am too sick to really digest or wrap my head around the fact that if they don't find a donor *tout suite*, I have about twelve days to live.

TEN

DECEMBER COMES, BUT INSTEAD OF COUNTING DOWN TO Christmas, my mother is counting days on ECMO. Friends and family send cards and gifts, and I am overwhelmed with love. My cousin Kirsten brings me a small purple Christmas tree for my room and a unicorn snow globe. My friend Lisa sends me a Prince ornament for the tree and a Prince blanket, which I promptly put over the boring hospital blanket. A dear friend from college, Brian, sends me an amazing Prince mug. A family friend, Sonya, sends a unicorn light to which she has added the famous opening line of Prince's song "Let's Go Crazy," making the ultimate mash-up of Team Glitter Unicorn and my Prince obsession. I adore every single unicorn and Prince-inspired gift. When Mom leaves the hospital each night, she looks up to see my room glowing from the soft purple lights of the tree sitting by the window.

I am in a stable, but extremely precarious and critical condition. It has now been almost three weeks since I've moved out of bed. In case you are wondering, yes, this means not even to going to the bathroom, which means bedpans. As it turns out, I will end up using bedpans for months. Have you ever had to use a bedpan as an immobile, middle-aged woman? It ranks right up there with getting a cavity filled.

Probably worse. I don't complain, because I am still alive. But, to be sure, it is a humiliating and humbling experience. As someone who is, as a psychic once described me, "fiercely independent" (my mother might counter with "stubborn"), having to rely on so many people for so many things—from my mother handling correspondence and being there every day, to doctors and nurses for big and small things like saving my life and wiping my ass—takes getting used to.

Finally, on December 3rd, we get some great news.

Mom's post in the Facebook group:

👍 🦄 *Well, all you wonderful Army of Team Glitter Unicorn, Aimee has allowed me the GREAT HONOR of letting you know that tonight they have reactivated her name on the double transplant list and her name goes to the top at their facility for her matches. We are happily and humbly thrilled, with a strong lump in our throats (a Mom thing).*

They are working hard to help get her strength back and some calories in her. The ECMO machine has done what they hoped but it is a mad scientist juggling of numbers to keep everything on a steady course. She is doing what she needs to do which is relax, rest, and now finally eat some food. But, most importantly, being engaged in the process, active in her medical care, and mentally visualize staying strong and resilient. Another wonderful step forward today and we will all help her get to her next goal, step by step!

Huge Hugs and thank you all for the love you have surrounded her and her family with. 🦄💜

Keep the magical medical miracles coming 😁💜

One hurdle down. I am reactivated on the list, and not a moment too soon. I am reactivated as a 1A—the direst of cases—and, as Mom says, I go straight to the top of the list. Mom has not left my side since October 9th. One thing this extravaganza has brought us is time together. Whether it can count as "quality time" is up for voracious debate. Still, I do delight in having Mom physically close. She doesn't know it, but her presence assuages some of my fears and anxiety in the way only moms can.

At this point, all the trepidation I once had about a transplant journey has long since dissipated under physical and mental exhaustion. I am beyond ready. I tell Mom that, while I am not at all scared about the surgery, I am apprehensive about the recovery. This worry would turn out to be a nice little case study of manifest destiny. Truly, thoughts are power.

✳

There's not much to do while we wait for "the call." We FaceTime with family. My brother and Dad visit. I have officially had to step away from my jobs. I email supervisors to keep them in the loop. I still have insurance through work, though that is contingent on me having a job and actually working. Another piece of the puzzle in this wild ride of life to figure out.

It's hard to write while lying in bed, and I don't have much of a passion for writing or reading at the moment. So, I watch "The Price is Right" on TV and devour Christmas movies like cookies. Every mental and physical ounce of me is preoccupied with surviving one day at a time. I'm not really depressed or super anxious, more like hopeful and a bit impatient, thanks to a finely crafted mental cocktail of optimism, faith, denial, and our family's brand of warped humor.

On December 11th, my mom posts the following in the Facebook group:

♥🐿️*Small update for this Wed. Been a bit of a 'rocky road' for the Poet today. Two steps forward, one step back, or peaks and valleys, take your pick. You know that old movie 'High Anxiety'? Well Aimee has the leading role and I know for certain she'd rather have just a walk on part in her own movie!!!! Deep breaths and hand holding for today with my girl. As you send her your good vibes, throw in a dose of Peace and calming energy to get her through this most excruciating wait she is feeling. This is hard . . .*

So, so hard. There is no telling how much longer the wait will be, but I have already exceeded the ECMO "time limit." It is a complete mindfuck of a paradox to be praying and wishing for a heart and liver while knowing that that means someone else has died. But wish and pray we do, trying to grapple with events as they come with all the grace and grit we can. They say good things come to those who have patience, but what if you have an expiration date?

✱

On December 12th, Dr. MacArthur, the transplant surgeon, comes in to deliver the news. There is an offer for a heart and liver, and it is determined to be a good match. I thrust my fist up in the air, John Bender-style. I am pumped and ready. I have every confidence and trust in Stanford and the teams of surgeons.

In the pre-op room, the anesthesiologist, Melissa, plays Prince music as I am prepped and we wait to hear that the organs are viable. At 7:35 PM, before I am wheeled away, Ralph takes a picture of Mom and me; I am lying on my silk pillowcase with my Prince blanket up to my neck. She is leaning over to give me a kiss. I honestly can't fathom what that must have been like for her, but I'm sure if she could have scrubbed in on the surgery, she would have. The sleepy meds are pushed through the IV before I make it to the OR, and I drift off into the most ultimate surrender I could ever conjure.

My brother arrives (for the second time in two weeks) a half an hour after I am rolled into surgery. My sister-in-law, Tiffany, was at the drug store when he called her, saying, "They found her a heart! You have to come home now and take me to the airport!" (Note: I now have the drug store receipt from when she got that call.)

At 8:45 PM, my mom gets the call that the organs are good and surgery is a go. Dr. MacArthur tells my mom, brother, and Ralph to go home and get some sleep. She gives him a look like, *Yeah, right, pal,* and instead, she, Ralph, and Johnny hang out in the small waiting area and hunker down to spend the night in the hospital.

✳

The surgery itself will take more than sixteen hours at least, during which I am given sixty units of blood. I imagine the surgeons' motions like expertly trained choreography. The heart team operates from one side of the table, and the liver team operates from the other. There are around fifteen people in the OR. In my mind, they perform an exquisite ballet of moving parts, precise procedures, nanosecond timing, and guts. The stage is blindingly bright, the beeping and sounding of monitors and alarms fill the air like a slightly agitated orchestra. There is heat, there is sweat, there is blood. Lots of blood. I have often thought of the downright gumption it must take to perform any surgery, let alone a transplant. Just swapping organs. No pressure.

Mom and Johnny couch surf around the hospital, looking for any dark corner to catch a few winks, while 6'5" Ralph makes due with the small loveseat/couch in my room. At 5:30 AM, they make their way down to the cafeteria and are first in line when it opens at 6:00 AM.

My mother writes in her journal on December 13th:

The gift of life was offered to Aimee on Thursday, December 12th, 2019. She was rolled into surgery at 7:25 with Ralph and I kissing her on her safe journey. I received a call at 8:45 from Fernando, the OR RN, to tell us the transplants would be a "Go" and they had received the call from the Stanford Heart and Liver transplant teams from Idaho that the donor organs where acceptable (perfect) and they would proceed with surgery there to remove them "en block" and then fly home to Stanford. At that point, Doctors JW MacArthur and liver surgeon Bonhem began Aimee's surgery here in Palo Alto.

The early morning hours of Friday, December 13ᵗʰ, the donor organs arrived and were placed in Aimee's body and at 3:33. The portal vein was unclamped and that would mean they started in her body on Friday the 13ᵗʰ at 3:33 am.

She officially has a second birthday! The enormity of this event will never be duplicated. I am so grateful to so many, first are Johnny, Tiffany, and Ralph — Lynn and Larry and a cast of hundreds of medical persons here and in TX, and hundreds of friends of Aimee's and our collective families here and all over the world.

✳

Once I am out of surgery and back in my room, one of the nurses, Jill, finds Mom, Ralph, Johnny, and Dad (who had flown in that morning). Scanning the group, she sizes up Mom as the one least likely to faint and says, "Mom, I will take you to see Aimee for a minute."

Mom describes the scene as a "madhouse," with a throng of people still working on me, surrounded by a mess of machines and equipment. There are lines and tubes coming out of every part of my body, lost in a pile of medical paraphernalia. My face and extremities are puffy, full of fluids, and my chest is Saran Wrapped like a bloody sandwich.

"There was so much blood," Mom says when I ask her about this later.

They are still working to stop some bleeding and give me another fifteen units of blood in the room. Almost immediately, Dr. MacArthur says to Mom:

"We're going to take her back down and get this bleeding under control." Eventually, they do get the bleeding under control.

My mom posts in the Glitter Unicorn Facebook group on December 13ᵗʰ:

For all of our "Team Unicorn" who really knows our dear Aimee, and the "road less traveled" she always takes… you know the one where you have two roads side by side, one asphalt and one dirt with rocks? Yep, Aimee is the gal who buys the Jeep and turns onto that bumpy road! She picks (I think she set us all up) 12/12 at 12:12 PM yesterday for me to sign consent forms and she has her new and improved organs delivered to her body on Freaky Friday the 13th!!!

So like her. So, her surgeon took her back into surgery for bleeding issues this afternoon and things went smoothly and bleeding slowed. They have not closed her incisions, as that would put too much pressure on new organs (something they must do often in multiple organ transplants). He said afterward she is doing well and to expect that she may go back to OR multiple times in the next few days. He asked us to let them do the worrying for her and we rest.

She will remain sedated for several days until bleeding has subsided and chest and abdomen are closed. She will not be aware of this turmoil around her. That comforts this Mom. The new organs are perfect and functioning now as they wished. They will keep her on ECMO for a few days to let her new heart and liver rest and not be overtaxed with all that they are throwing at her right now.

I am sure Aimee would question my burdening you all with such great details, but you have all been on this journey with us and deserving of the truth she is facing and why your strength of positive love and prayer is so needed! It's not for the faint of heart and this child I know has never given up. She picked you all to join us and we have gained Peace in knowing you are standing with us.

One day this is going to all make sense, but for tonight I will be happy for the moment!

Hang in there with us!

The numbers seven and thirteen have always been my favorite numbers and I absolutely love the fact that I receive my new organs on Friday the 13th. Though Friday the 13th conjures up specific pop culture images surrounding Jason and the mask that are indelibly etched into every Gen Xer's brain, I have still always loved the number thirteen. And the universal symmetry of 12/12 and 12:12 is too undeniably obvious to ignore. Twelve zodiac signs. Twelve months in a year. Twelve apostles. Each month, each zodiac, represents a new cycle of growth and transformation.

As Mom says, the first few days after surgery are incredibly delicate. To my end, I do not remember these days; instead, I rely on my mother's journal for a glimpse into this time.

On December 18th, my mom writes in her journal about the past six days:

The pitfalls. Surgery — massive bleeding (Friday the 13th). Over 60 units of blood and other products given in OR. Then in her room for 4 and half hours and 15 more units, plus plasma and platelets and other blood products and was returned to OR because of bleeding. Returned to OR on Sat 12/14 for a wash out and check for bleeding. Only 1 unit of blood was given this day. Sunday was a hold steady day. Monday 12/16 they told us they planned to take her to OR for wash out and perhaps close her chest and abdomen. She was finally taken to OR around 2-3am on Thursday 12/17 and finished at 5am.

In a Facebook post to the group, my mom writes about the surgery and the following days:

I have been waiting to post updates as so much changes day to day and hour to hour! To say this girl loves the "adventurous" side of life is a given! But she is a warrior personified!!! She may be small, but she is mighty in spirit and so far resilient as heck! Here is a brief timeline of the past week.

Thursday 12/12 taken to surgery

Friday 12/13 out of surgery around 11 am and returned to OR for bleeding around 3 pm. Over the course of surgery and in her room before she went back to surgery for the bleeding Aimee received over 75 units of whole blood and also numerous other blood products! Over 9 times what her body would hold. (Please donate blood 💧 if you can)

Saturday 12/14 returned to OR for washing out of the entire surgical site, but received only 1 unit of blood and no more bleeding.

Sunday 12/15 was a hold steady day

Monday 12/16 was told they would finally close her chest and abdomen which was a very big deal. Finally got her into OR in the middle of the night early morning and I believe she was completed by 5 AM Tuesday morning.

Tuesday 12/17. Steady and watching her organs function now that they were sutured closed in her body. Overnight Tuesday night they started her on gentle continuous dialysis to remove excess fluid that they had had to throw at her. They had told us she would most likely have this temporarily at some point and that line was placed in her during transplant.

Wednesday 12/18 her face was much skinnier so dialysis was working and we were told around noon that when an OR was available, they would take her back to surgery to remove her from the ECMO machine.

She was finally rolled into OR around 8 PM last night and I received a call from her transplant surgeon at 1:30 AM this morning that she had been successfully removed from ECMO and organs working fine. She is still sedated and very very slowly coming to slight moments of consciousness but remains with breathing tube. They will want to remove that in the next day or so but there is a good chance they will do a tracheostomy in her throat for a while to assist her to breathe, as she is soooo weakened by being flat in bed for weeks now. I have only given you a penny's worth of what has transpired and have forgotten more than I even can remember.

One of her ICU attending told me she is making tiny steps in the right direction, but this will be a slow process and bumpy.

My one sweet bright moment and only one so far was yesterday around 6 PM, she seemed a bit lucid and when the nurse told her to look to her left side that her Mom was there she smiled at me a couple of times and nodded her head. I want more of those moments!!!!

Please forgive me for not posting more but the roller coaster ride is REAL and very hard to give accurate information as it changes nearly before I finish a post! 🖤

Love you all for your continued prayers and loving energy you are sending her. I know she had been humbled by your generosity of loving friendship!!! Keep up the good fight, and one last nugget you will get a kick out of! Yesterday when we had that moment of connection her nurse told her that the House had voted for 2 articles of Impeachment and she raised her eyes and smiled!!! 🖤🐎 *XO*

PS... In my haste to get a post up, I failed miserably in saying thank you to some very important people (besides all the incredible medical professionals we are grateful for).

To Ralph for his enormous love and care for Me, Aimee, and Johnny! To Johnny for the great love he has shown his sister and his flying in at a moment's notice twice! To Tiffany for loving all of us and holding down the fort at home with 4 young children AND Aimee's 15-year-old, 3-legged pup Elfie who now wears a cast on her one good front leg! To her Dad for flying up from SoCal to Larry and Lynn North (Aimee's aunt and uncle) who have taken us all in, fed us, loved on us, and made the days a tiny slice of normal. Our hearts are grateful.

If it takes a village to raise a child, then it takes a city to uplift a transplant family.

ELEVEN

IT'S THE SEASON OF GOODWILL, AND NOTHING SAYS miracle like receiving a heart and liver when virtually on the brink of the point of no return. Now begins the slow and arduous mountain climb of recovery. On December 18th, Mom writes in her journal:

More alert this Thursday and great in the afternoon as she was able to nod, smile, and interact with the breathing tube in. Overnight Wednesday into Thursday, ECMO was removed.

I don't have any recollection of these first days post-surgery. Because of swelling and bleeding and wanting to make sure the heart and liver are responding, my chest and abdomen are kept "open" for a few days post-op. Basically, they Saran Wrap me until I am ready to be sutured up for good.

I have to take a minute here and talk about the use and removal of the ECMO. I am told that I am the first patient at Stanford to undergo the use of ECMO as a bridge to a heart and liver transplant and SURVIVE post-surgery. This is so ground-breaking and extraordinary that one of the Residents,

Sumeet Viakunth, and a few others, publish the following in an article called, "Extracorporeal Membrane Oxygenator as a Bridge to Heart-Liver En Bloc Transplant in a Fontan Patient,"[9] in *JTCVS Techniques* journal about a year later:

We report here the first successful use of VA-ECMO in an adult failing Fontan patient as a bridge to heart-liver transplant. Although VA-ECMO has been used in failing Fontan patients as a bridge to VAD and heart transplant alone, it has not been used as a bridge to heart-liver en bloc transplant. The major concerns for ECMO in Fontan patients are achieving adequate venous drainage and ensuring afterload is not too high on the single ventricle when trying to achieve satisfactory ECMO flows. A straightforward cannulation strategy of femoral artery and vein allowed for adequate venous drainage and support of hemodynamics. ECMO afforded this patient additional time to overcome an acute insult on top of her failing Fontan physiology while preserving end organ perfusion, ultimately allowing her to remain a candidate for transplantation. As more Fontan patients reach adulthood and start to fail, institution of peripheral ECMO remains a viable option to stabilize and bridge these patients to transplant.

Aren't science and technology amazing? I owe my life to science and technology. I owe my spirit to the universe, which I choose to believe always arcs toward benevolence. I believe we are spiritual beings inhabiting a human body for a time. For me, this lifetime came with a bit of heavy-duty body maintenance.

I am told I was awake and conscious during these days, but I don't remember any of it. I do know my mom and Ralph were with me every day. My brother returned to Texas after a few days, and Dad returned to Palm Springs, but I don't recall saying goodbye. Closing in on the first week post-transplant, my mother writes in her journal on December 20th:

A good "numbers" day, but not for understanding and

interaction. They had the ventilator off for 5-6 hours and she is/was breathing on her own. They did take her for a CT scan because her white blood count is up to 31,000, so infection somewhere. She was very exhausted today and is not sleeping at night with all the steroids.

Then on December 21st:

Called as I was driving to hospital as they want to take her to surgery to remove breathing tube and place a trach so that they can get her to breathe better and move and get her to sit up. She is somewhat responsive to me and acknowledged me and nodded to a few questions.

December 21st is when I start to have any real post-op memories. I wake up with the face of a wonderful nurse shining down on me like soft sunlight. She looks so serene that for a split second, I don't know if I am still earthside. She is smiling and looks and feels a bit like an angel. Then, I notice her name tag says "Maria." My first thought is, *Did I have the surgery yet?*

"Is the surgery over?" I ask Maria.

She smiles. "It's all over."

"What day is it?" I ask.

"The twenty-first."

I am shocked that I have seemingly been "unconscious" for a week. But I am thrilled the surgery is over and that I am still, to be honest, alive. I start to slowly become more responsive and more coherent. It is also around this time where the ICU delirium starts to set in. In an article written by Dr. Haleema Yezdani, ICU delirium is defined as ". . .a condition, or rather, a complication of hospitalization in the intensive care unit. It is characterized by a set of symptoms ranging from mere confusion to agitation. It can also be called acute brain dysfunction of critically ill patients," according to medindia.net.

We'll get to the fun ICU delirium in a minute, but first, doctors decide to remove the breathing tube in favor of a tracheostomy tube. In a Facebook post to the group on December 22nd, my mom writes:

Tiny update: Aimee just got back from the OR and they removed the breathing tube from her mouth and put in a tracheostomy temporarily. She was breathing on her own for about 6 hrs yesterday at one stretch and again before OR and also now. The tracheostomy will allow her to be able to sit up and eventually to a chair, and if she needs oxygen, then she will have it to help her expand her lungs (remember she has been flat on her back for over 3 weeks). One of the several potholes she is navigating at present is not being able to get sleep. The combination of many of the drugs they must use post-transplant for a while keep you awake and "wire" you. Even with a few different sleeping medications the last 3 nights, she isn't sleeping. She needs rest to heal, but also must have these meds 😩 Cray Cray!!!! But as I sit here looking at her sweet face without the tubes in her mouth, I rejoice that another tiny step was taken in the right direction today. 😊

Was looking for pictures to show her nurse what "our" girl looked like prior to surgery and came across her DL pic I had taken and took a large breath because there was her red heart DONOR sticker at the bottom right! The enormity of what that symbolizes today verses the unconscious act that I have always checked the box struck me hard.

We are so so grateful and in awe. We are still deep in the forest on her journey and looking for sunlight! The trail may be very long, but we have your love and energy to keep us going forward! Take time out to celebrate 🎉 yourselves this weekend and know you are in my thoughts daily and in Aimee's dreams at present 💜 Hugs 🖤🦄

To fill you in, having a trach means being hooked up to a ventilator 24/7. The ventilator is a huge machine that is plugged in to the wall and lives on left side of my bed. Its purpose is to deliver oxygen to the lungs while removing carbon dioxide. Since my lungs were on the weaker side even before surgery, the ventilator helps with lung function, and is, for the most part, a fairly typical part of heart/liver transplants, but a side-effect that we had not even thought about.

The trach feels like wearing a choker necklace with a long, flimsy plastic tube coming out of it. You can't talk without a special speaking valve. And it takes practice to work with the speaking valve. While on the ventilator, it must go everywhere you go; it becomes a mechanical appendage. The Respiratory Therapists are specially trained to work with patients on the ventilator. Also, one annoying thing about being on a ventilator is that you're still making saliva, but you can't spit it up or really swallow it, so at least three or four times a day, when you need it, the nurse will temporarily detach the tube, push a suction device down the trach hole, extend it down into your esophagus and suck. And yes, it is just as unpleasant as it sounds. I always brace for the gag I know is coming.

Since I can't talk, Mom arms me with a legal pad and pen so I can write things down. She also becomes an expert lip reader. Of this day, the 22nd, she writes in her journal:

Another good numbers day and spontaneous breathing most all day. Responded to me and her father in late morning. Krissy and Ralph here at 2pm. (Which I actually do remember) *At times she seems alert and furrows her brow, then other times she seems very fuzzy. Tried to tell us something but couldn't understand. 2 nurses taking care of her – Avita and Edden. Not in pain. Turned off sedation and anxiety meds. Calm night's sleep is not very good – 3 hours last eve. White blood count over 40,000 – what is going on?*

For context, a normal WBC is between 4,000 and 11,000, which means I have a raging infection somewhere. I am aware that it is almost Christmas, and I keep my purple tree lit 24/7. Friends and family send cards and Mom tapes all of them on the wall, building a beautiful mural of peace and love. My dad visits again, as does Ralph's daughter, Krissy. Although I am making incremental progress, it is a very touch-and-go period. Things change quickly and often. But there are smatterings of delicate, lovely moments, as my mother writes in Team Glitter Unicorn Facebook group on December 30th:

A wonderful treat again today😊 Claudia, one of the harp players came in and played a few tunes "Leaves of Gold" and "Somewhere Over the Rainbow" and others. So lovely❤

Mini update would be that she is hungry, but can't have anything yet.

Asked for a cheeseburger! My kind of girl! White Blood cell count coming down nicely and that reflects infection issue. Trying to dissolve blood clots in chest with clot-buster fluids, doing a procedure later today to drain some fluids, etc, etc, etc. Watching Forrest Gump at present after Castaway earlier!

Just two girls hanging out watching flicks, one gets sedation and the other one wants some!!!!! 😴😴😴. Mini steps and more mini steps seems to be our course😅

May the last day of the old year tomorrow be cherished and appreciated, and our dreams for the New Year be eventually fulfilled. 🤩

Hugs from A & A 😊😊🙏❤

I can definitely empathize with Dorothy from *The Wizard of Oz* singing that showstopper. She is pining for a place where troubles melt away like candy while desperately wanting to fly high into the sky. The ultimate musical escape ballad. Me too, girl. Me too.

It's also true that I beg—through Mom's lipreading translations—Dr. MacArthur for a cheeseburger, even though I know I can't have one and I know he can't let me have one. The feeding tube hanging from my nose is making my nose ache and it's just plain annoying. Sigh. As the poet A.E. Stallings says: "Nothing is more permanent than the temporary."

On New Year's Eve, dozens of friends and family flood the Facebook Team Glitter Unicorn group with "Happy New Year" messages. And you know what? It is. The group has become—besides a place for Mom to update everyone all at once—an amazing collection of Unicorn, Prince, and Paris posts, which is exactly my vibe. While I feel a modicum of moroseness about being in the hospital on New Year's Eve, I am buoyed and uplifted by these well wishes.

✳

Now, back to our regularly scheduled post-op side-effect: ICU delirium. Mine manifests in some of the most bizarre and vivid dreams I have ever had. These dreams feel and seem so real that it sometimes takes me awhile to figure out what was real and what was not. The dreams are either hilarious or, more often, utterly terrifying:

Dream 1: I dream that I am in the hospital post-transplant (as I am) and I am pregnant. I think that my mother is going to be livid with me, but she is over the moon. She even makes a gushy Facebook post, saying something to the effect of "even though this is not the ideal situation, we are thrilled and looking forward to meeting Baby Mackovic!" And one of my best friend's comments on her Facebook post, saying "Congratulations!!!" It feels so real that, a day or two later, hand to Universe, I ask my mom if I'm pregnant. She bursts out laughing: "No, honey." And, no, no idea who the father would have been.

Dream 2: I dream that I am an extremely disruptive patient in a mental institution. I escape into the rain, but am soon caught. I am taken to a huge, one-room ward with rows and rows of women laying side by side in a huge bed, cramped in like sardines. We are all outcasts. I make another disturbance, and they throw me out in the rain again. I am then taken to an isolation cell.

Dream 3: I dream that one of my favorite nurses, Dorothy, offers to tattoo me right in my hospital room. It feels like it is taking place in real time, so this is only weeks post-surgery. She says, "Well, Aimee, we've got some time before your next procedure, why don't I give you a tattoo?" She then pulls out all her tattooing equipment and starts setting up. She decides I should get a tattoo on my back hip, so she props me up on my side. Now, I have three tattoos in real life, and the funny thing to me is that the real Dorothy is, besides being an awesome nurse, an incredibly sweet, nurturing woman and not necessarily the kind of person you think about when you think of tattoo artists. It is by far the most hilarious delirium I have and still makes me giggle. The next day, I write out a short explanation of the dream for my mom and Dorothy and we all roar with some much-needed laughter.

Dream 4: I dream that my father has come to town to see me. But before he comes to see me, he goes to his hotel and gets roaring drunk, which is absolutely the last thing he would do. He comes to the hospital and ends up getting into a fistfight with a nurse or doctor in my room. The other person is arrested. I am worried sick that the hospital is going to press charges against Dad, even though he *was* the one who instigated the fight. Even in this dream-slash-nightmare, Mom somehow knows of the whole thing. She comes in the next morning in the dream, leans down to me and smiles. "No charges," she says, smiling broadly, and I am flooded with relief.

Until the next dream.

Dream 5: I dream that a nurse gets wind that it was my dad who caused trouble. He gets down in my face and asks, "He's your dad? He's the reason my uncle is in jail." He and a few other nurses proceed to strap me down to the bed. They then start rolling me around the hospital, outside, everywhere, even through an outdoor promenade with shops and restaurants where people are dining. The nurses are part of a secret society of nurses who are anti-nurses. They are cruel and mentally and physically abusive. They have put me in wrist and ankle restraints and mock me to my face while parading me. They are playing some sort of twisted mind games with me. My defense is to go catatonic; I don't respond and don't engage. After what feels like a very long time, they leave me in a cavernous, dark abandoned shopping mall. My mom and family are on the other side of a huge, locked door. I can hear them and, now alone, try calling out to her, to no avail.

Dream 6: I dream I live in a nice, spacious apartment on top of a football stadium. There is an elevator that will take me straight down to a Prince concert. A random couple comes into the apartment and tells me it is their apartment. Then, Mack and Sally Brown (family friends—he is a famous college football coach) come in and tell the couple, "No, this is Aimee's apartment." (Thanks, Browns!) A bunch of football players in various team jerseys come and hang out in the living room, watching various games on the huge television as if they do this all the time. This delirium is the least complicated dream to interpret and is completely comical. If it's not apparent, I love football and Prince.

By far the most terrifying dream is the one where I watch Ralph die as I am shackled with wrist and ankle restraints. I am at a fancy, but darkly lit party, in my hospital bed (because even in the delirium—or perhaps because of it—I can't escape the bed) and one of the servers is actually a nurse from the hospital, moonlighting. She absolutely does not like me for some reason. Presiding over the party from a balcony is a gorgeous, but cruel, woman who is dressed a bit like royalty. She doesn't speak, but has power over everyone and everything. Ralph is there, trying to advocate for my release. With a look, the woman slowly sucks the life force out of him. I am crushed and wailing. Still dreaming (but believing I am now fully awake and coherent) I am then back in the hospital and overhear my mother sitting on the small couch under the windows that look out. She is on the phone, overwhelmingly sad, but stoic in talking to someone and making arrangements.

In a beat, it is the next day in real life, but this feels indistinguishable from the delirium, and I am so startled by this dream and convinced that it was real, that when Ralph walks into the hospital room alive and strong, I am speechless.

TWELVE

NEW YEAR. NEW ROLLERCOASTER. THE FIRST WEEK OF January is intense. My mother writes in her journal around January 4th:

December 24-January 3 Very up and down and pretty scary. Dr. Charles Hall on [rotations] *that week of New Year's Eve and Melissa (anesthesia transplant resident) both very concerned by the ways things were going. Lungs full of old blood. Bronchoscopy done. White blood count up. Then either changed or started some steroids that are produced by adrenal glands and things improved. One of her kidneys (right) has a hematoma cap* [small pocket of blood] *on it so it was damaged in surgery.*

As Mom notes, the doctors do a bronchoscopy to look at my lungs and find them full of old blood, which will require medical intervention, though it is not an absolute emergency. They start to try to get me out of the bed and sitting in a recliner chair. Every other day or so, they use a Hoyer lift (think body sling) to get me out of the bed and move me over to the chair to sit upright. This sling is an ingenious contraption allowing nurses to move otherwise immobile patients in and out of bed without hurting the patient or themselves. The body sling is slipped under me, then the four corners are hooked to a device mounted on the ceiling, which is connected to a track on the ceiling, allowing the sling to slide back and forth across the room. Slowly, I am scooped up and gently folded in like a flower, then slid over to the chair and lowered down into the chair. I call it the "shortest flight ever."

✳

What Mom and I are beginning to comprehend is that recovery is going to be painstakingly slower and harder than we anticipated. Riding the waves of ups and down requires extreme emotional calisthenics; it is the most physically and emotionally challenging journey we have been on, when it comes to my heart journey. We are going to have to learn how to surf these waves. My mother writes in a Facebook post to the group on January 7th:

Hello lovely family and friends 😊. As the warm sun is setting outside the window, I wait for Aimee to get back to her room from the OR. Two procedures that have been planned and normal. First is heart biopsy and the other is basically clearing out of the right pleural cavity so lungs can function more normally and then get off the tracheostomy eventually.

Yesterday Aimee was moved from the J236 room to J420! 420 has such a nice ring to it don't ya think?😊. She is requiring a little less care, so this is a step in the right direction. Another mini step forward on this marathon 🖤😊. I counted up some days today... so far 105 consecutive days. 15 at Dell Children's in Austin, flown to Stanford, 51 on 5 different floors prior to ECMO, 39 in room J236 from ECMO thru transplant, and now 1 in J 420. Whew, and we aren't done yet.

Yesterday there was a moment that was so lovely, but so profound when one of our very favorite doctors, and reason we are here, came to check in on Aimee and said, "You know Aimee you are no longer a congenital heart defect patient!" Yikes 😱

And that's true. After 44 years of that mindset, and filling out forms that way, it kind of took my breath away 😵 In a good way 😄 . I think Aimee got her money's worth out of that sweet old heart ❤️ The hard patient work begins in earnest. Thank you all for taking this ride with us 🦄💜❤️

Namaste

When one of our favorites, Dr. Lui, tells us that I'm not longer his patient, because I am "no longer a congenital heart defect" patient, it hits us. Oh, right! New heart! No more defect! The poignancy of this moment takes our breath away. After forty-four years, I now have a new-to-me defect-free heart. In truth, I don't think of the heart as mine. It's not mine. It is on permanent loan from a selfless soul I desperately wish I could thank in person. Her recycled parts have allowed me, and my family, a second chance. There is not a day when I don't think about my donor and wonder about her. The only thing I can do now is live with purpose.

✳

Enough mush, back to blood. So, about this blood in the lungs. The "clearing out of the right pleural cavity (lung)" is necessary due to some pleural effusion, or, in layman's terms, fluid in the lining of the lung. I come out of the procedure with a few more tubes in my right side, which are removed after a few days. I am not in terrible pain, but it is not exactly comfortable.

The days are spent working with different teams on rehabilitation, such as physical therapy and speech therapy. I am, at first, resistant to physical therapy. My limbs feel like cement and even shifting myself in bed is an extreme chore. They still use the sling to get me from the bed to the chair. I am encouraged by doctors and nurses to spend a few hours each day in the chair sitting upright, as even the simple act of sitting helps build strength. But right now, I feel weak, and frustrated at my lack of mobility and the fact that I still have to use a bedpan. I am trying to listen to my body, which is screaming: *just give us a sec!* while also trying to listen to the doctors and nurses who are, rightfully, pushing me.

And, as far as that whole hematoma on the kidney thing goes, we are told that the kidneys are the most diva-like of organs, and that if they don't wake up after six months, they most likely won't. In the meantime, however, I will require intermittent dialysis. So, on January 9th, they place a tunnel catheter for dialysis, which is necessary due to end-stage kidney disease, a byproduct of the intense surgery. Unfortunately, kidney failure after a liver transplant is not uncommon. It is estimated that between 20% to 80% of liver transplant patients will develop chronic kidney disease, ultimately leading to a kidney transplant, according to a study published on PubMed.com called, "Chronic kidney disease after liver transplantation: Recent evidence," by Fabrizio Fabrizi and others.[10]

Kidney failure can occur almost immediately after transplant or down the line. My understanding is that a heart transplant (let alone a heart/liver transplant) is exponentially harder on the body than other transplants, leading to almost immediate kidney failure. Kidney failure can also occur down the line due to the transplant medications that patients will have to take for life.

The dialysis port is snuggled under my left clavicle, right above my boob. Dialysis is going to be three times a week for about three-and-a-half hours. The process itself is not painful or particularly unpleasant; I'm just hooked up to a machine and have to sit there. Like I could go anywhere, anyway! Besides cleaning the blood of impurities, dialysis takes off excess fluid, which is bad for the new heart. Because the surgeons had given me so much blood and so many fluids during and since surgery—more than seventy-five units of blood in one day alone!—I am still retaining too much fluid. My feet and hands are extremely puffy with water weight. Every time they take two liters off, I puff back up again. A reinflating flesh balloon.

The sessions themselves are fairly boring and time-consuming. The technician wheels two large machines into the room and plugs them to the wall. I'm jazzed up with a blood pressure cuff on the arm, which I usually have on anyways, and a pulse oximeter on a finger. The blood pressure cuff is set to take a blood pressure reading every fifteen minutes during the three-and-a-half-hour treatment, since dialysis can cause a drop in blood pressure. I am given medication through the machine to prevent this. The technician then swabs the catheter (and me) down with alcohol. Sterilization is especially important, since my catheter line goes straight to my heart and any kind of infection would be a huge snag, to put it mildly. Masks are put on me and the technician. After that, the catheter is hooked up to two lines, one line for taking my blood out of my body to the machine, where it is fed to the machine through one line, cleaned, then returned as clean blood through the other line.

As with everything in life, there are tradeoffs.

THIRTEEN

"SO, IT'S GOING TO FEEL LIKE YOU'RE DROWNING," SAYS Sandra, the speech therapist, "but just relax and try to clear your throat."

She is working with me on using the Passy Muir valve, otherwise called a speaking valve. It is a small device placed over the trach opening at the throat, which allows the user to talk. I have, for weeks now, been relegated to scribbling questions and comments on a yellow legal pad I keep within arm's reach. I am not an overly talkative person by nature, but isn't it the rule that you don't miss something until it's gone?

"Ready?" she asks. I nod, but am not prepared for when she places it on. Instantly, I feel fifteen feet underwater. I can't breathe and my pulse quickens. My eyes bug out like a cartoon as I try to sputter and clear my throat, but I can't quite do it. It is a wild sensation and paradoxical to feel like I'm simultaneously submerged under water and sitting in a hospital bed on dry land. Instinctively, my arms flail.

"Try to clear your throat" she says. I try, but it feels insanely hard to do so.

She watches me and waits about five seconds before she takes it out. I take a minute to regain compose and get my breath back.

I try again, this time managing to at least try clearing my throat. Not totally successful, but better than last time.

"Better!" she says. "Okay, let's try once more."

I try again with a bit more success. I am able to clear my throat and no longer feel like I'm under water. She prompts me to say something, so I look at Mom and squeak out, "I love you, Mom."

Cue all of us getting pee-pee eyed, as Ralph would say. Happy tears.

The next day, I work with the valve again. Mom and I FaceTime my brother and Ralph. I also manage to walk with a walker and the wonderful physical therapist, Ben, to the door and back. There is a video of me with my walker and all the machines—IV pole, trach, catheter, and chest tube bags hanging off—taking the ten steps to the door and promptly turning around. My shoulders are up by my ears and I am white knuckling the walker, but it is a good day. Mom writes this in a Facebook post on January 11th:

All in all, through the ups and downs of this week, Aimee is giving it a pink lip smile tonight! Sunday has been a good rest day for her (wanted and needed) as Monday will arrive soon. PT and OT, Speech and Swallow Specialist, Dialysis, perhaps another tube removed but perhaps another will be placed in the left lung this week. It's body-part Bingo and Aimee has just about filled her whole card! Our anatomy course continues and we are now tops in our class or close 🍪🍪 We wish you all a good and healthy week ahead as we try to "kick butt" here! 🖤 🐿

This journey is about learning how to cha-cha as I move forward through the setbacks. It is a slow, grueling process. I am never bitter or angry about my situation; I mean, there is nothing I can do about it, and I know that stewing and being angry at the universe isn't going help get me out of this hospital any faster.

That isn't to say that I don't have down days. There are many, many down days. There comes a point where even the most positive of attitudes is maligned by reality. The reality is that this is an extremely arduous recovery, physically and emotionally. Yes, there is still hope and pushing through, but instead of being my usual "Pollyanna" self, I have to meet myself right where I am at this moment, which is frustrated. Fucking frustrated.

One thing that helps is taking ownership of the things I can control and trying not to let the other things which I cannot control rot my brain like maggots. One thing I can control: work on walking. One thing I cannot control: scheduling. When you are an inpatient having two to four different procedures a week that require scheduling (such as caths, x-rays, etc.), the hospital schedules you on the contingency that emergencies don't pop up. And emergencies always pop up. This is in addition to outpatients who also already have procedures scheduled. So, scheduling can be tricky. Since I am a planner and like to "schedule my day" (even in a freaking hospital!), I get easily frustrated when procedures or therapies are delayed by hours, or even rescheduled to the next day, especially when I have been NPO (no feeding tube) since midnight the night before, as per pre-procedure protocol. This means I miss out on whatever little nutrition I could have gotten. And this happens multiple times, no real fault of Stanford's. They are just doing their jobs and doing them splendidly. But still, it is a source of frustration that I, and my mother, have to work through.

Another proactive thing we can do: my mother and I ask to have a meeting with all the teams. A family can never really emotionally prepare for a transplant, and my mother and I had had visions of fairly smooth sailing with maybe light wind. But this? This is tsunami-level winds. We had no frame of reference to anticipate how rough it was really going to be. So, after navigating the first almost four-week, post-transplant period with some major potholes, we ask to have a meeting with all the teams—kidney, heart, liver, infectious disease, the janitors.

Mom does the talking for us, as I scribble comments or questions. Both of us come out of that meeting with a better understanding of the upcoming recovery journey. We learn that a double heart/liver transplant is often the toughest to recover from. We have a better idea of how to manage our own expectations. We have to let go of our idea of what we thought the recovery was going to be like in order to simply deal with the situation as it is currently. Easier said than done, but it helps me shift my mentality from: "Why am I not getting better faster?" to "This is where I am at today. What can I do to move forward?"

The good news is that the heart and liver are working perfectly, and every heart biopsy so far has come back with zero trace of rejection. They confirm that I am making progress, albeit slowly. Their job is to keep on top of any issues that come up; my job is to try and do as much physical therapy and speech therapy as I can. I'll admit that, in the beginning, my motivation is pretty pitiful. I still feel physically depleted, and even just moving to the side of the bed feels like scaling Kilimanjaro, not to mention actually getting to my feet and walking. But, like Billy Murray says, baby steps.

It is around this time where, just to add to the fun, I start experiencing some gastro-intestinal issues and start bleeding slightly from my nether parts, so we add a gastroenterologist to the team. This sets off a chain of events I like to call the Let's See How Many Procedures We Can Do On Aimee-palooza. There are abdominal MRIs, which only show that there is bleeding, but not where it's coming from. So, it's on to the really fun stuff—like a colonoscopy. Yay! Said no one ever.

The gastroenterologist wants to do a colonoscopy and endoscopy to pinpoint where the bleeding is coming from. The endoscopy involves the inserting of a small camera down my throat, down into the digestive tract, while under sedation. No biggie. Now, if you've ever had a colonoscopy, you know the procedure itself is a breeze—you're put under sedation for what seems like a minute, and then you're awake again. It's the preparation that's a bitch. The idea is to look at the digestive tract from the top and bottom to find the source of the bleeding.

Later that night, the nurse, almost apologetically, comes in with three huge jugs of the Golightly, which is a drink meant to, to be frank, make you go to the bathroom until you're as clean as a whistle in preparation for the procedure. I take one sip of the Golightly and gag. *This isn't going to happen,* I think, and scribble down a note on a notepad that says as much.

Instead, he gives me a drug through the IV once an hour that does the same thing. Perfect. But that is only half the battle. Keep in mind, I have been using a bedpan and needing the help of nurses to go to the bathroom since November. Besides being weak, I am tethered with multiple IV lines and the ventilator, so getting out of the bed and to the bathroom (especially quickly) is not an option. Each time I have to go to the bathroom is an ordeal for myself and the nurses. It is a lengthy process requiring two people. First, pull the covers down to my feet. Then, I am rolled to one side by one nurse, while the other maneuvers the cold, plastic bedpan underneath my tush. After I am done, I am again rolled to one side, then suspended there as the bedpan is removed and I am wiped down from that side. Then, I am rolled to the other side to finish the wiping. This is also when they change out the soiled pad underneath my tush for a clean one. Finally, I am rolled onto my back and covered up again.

And then, just when you think it can't get any more farcical—my mother's journal entry from Wednesday, January 22nd says:

Given Golightly for colonoscopy (didn't happen). Given pooping meds all night long, did not sleep. Finished bag of Golightly just after noon. Dr. Goel came in early afternoon and said they would not do her procedure today because she wasn't cleaned out enough. Aimee slept until awakened at 3:50pm to walk with Ben. Then she sat in chair until 6:45. Will start Golightly again to run overnight and try to get her cleaned out and do both procedures in the AM. Tried to pin down on "scheduled" time tomorrow and that she not be an "add on."

Dr. Goel told Aimee and me that it would be first thing in the morning! Momma Bear is hot. Asked them to find out a time for Aimee, as she will also need dialysis tomorrow. No trach collar today. No speech [therapy] since last week. Golightly started after 8pm.

It is a rough couple of days on my body, which is bleeding and being rubbed raw from the constant wiping. But there are many times where the nurses are busy when I am in need of a bedpan, so I work out a system where I hike my gown up to my hips, making sure I'm not lying on it, push the covers down towards my ankles and go on said pad resting under my butt. *shrug emoji* Real talk. I agree; it is gross and totally undignified. But isn't life sometimes? All I can say is that I owe a huge debt to the nurses on duty those couple of nights. Bless you Rangel, Leah, Dorothy, Gilbert, Bridgette, Grette, and so many others.

A new dawn brings fresh opportunity. Mom's journal entry on Thursday, January 23rd:

Golightly is going until 11am or so. Now they are saying they will do both procedures [colonoscopy and endoscopy] at bedside after 1pm. Aimee is now bleeding in trach suction tube and a lot in bedpan. She is worried and concerned. She is exhausted from little sleep for last 2 nights of pooping. No trach collar. Kidney team now says no dialysis today, will wait till tomorrow. She says she can't wiggle all her toes on left foot. Coloring on bottom of feet is a bit purple again. Procedures done at bedside starting around 1:35pm. Dr. Goel and Dr. Zo gave consent at 3pm for them to insert a pill camera at the top of small bowel and it will video for next 12 hours and hopefully find the bleed as nothing could be found in either direction so must be in an area not seen yet. Tolerated well.

Sometimes, like life, medicine is a case of experimentation. It is a marvel to me that they can insert a camera the size of a pill into the top of my bowels and have it record images. Like, does the camera get WIFI in there?! These procedures go off smoothly, but still don't offer any true answers. Or rather, the doctors don't see anything causing this on-and-on bleeding.

On January 24th, I write my first and only journal entry while in the hospital in a newly gifted notebook. The cover of the notebook is a colorful unicorn, meant to uplift. Well, it didn't quite work to cheer me up that day. Oscillating between gratitude, supreme frustration, trying to stay positive, and the absolute sucky-ness of the whole situation, I write the following:

I am really frustrated but ok. I want to get back to living. I hate the trach and it is really hard to walk. I underestimated the whole thing. I know I am making good progress, but it is going to be a long road. I want out of here and I know that day will come. I miss my dog and friends, but am so grateful for my mom. I'm trying to get stronger faster, but it is hard. I never thought I would have to learn to walk again. I'm grateful for Stanford. I look forward to going to Mom's house. I love it there. I am grateful for UT and Keiser [employers] who have been amazing.

I want to get back to living. I want to travel. I want to do yoga. I want my old life back. I know it will come, maybe not as fast as I would like. Some days are better than others. I feel confined and I don't like that. I know this is a marathon, but it is truly the hardest thing I have ever done.

I want to get back to writing. I feel bad not writing, but I don't think I can right now. I feel behind in my writing career, though I'm not really. I want to be in Poetry and The New Yorker. My chest feels tight and my breathing feels shallow, though they always say my numbers look good. Lying in bed most of the day is hell. I am sick of procedures and tests. I've lost count.

One day at a time. I'm learning that the recovery process is going to be anything but linear. Like any kind of upward-ly-trending graph, if you look at it from a distance, you can easily see steady growth, but when you get closer, you see all the actual pitfalls and valleys in between the peaks. I am also learning that the less attached and flustered I get with the everyday ups and down and, instead, try to think long term, the more manageable the emotional quagmire becomes. Still, this does not happen overnight and, in the age of instant gratification, takes a tremendous amount of internal work and soul maintenance.

FOURTEEN

"AIMEE, IT'S OKAY TO HAVE A BAD DAY," SAYS DR. MACARTHUR. Until he says this, I had not known how much I needed and wanted to hear that. I (and my whole family) have spent so much energy and focus on staying positive, that I had forgotten that admitting how sucky things are at the moment can also serve a purpose. What's that saying? Meet yourself where you're at.

After a month of molasses-like progress and dozens of procedures, he knows that I am grasping for some good news and motivation. I am, more than I've even been, worried about my condition. I have developed a bad habit of watching my blood pressure and saturation monitors like a hawk.

"Turn the monitors around," Dr. MacArthur says. "Don't look at them. We are not going to let anything happen to you. As far as your heart and liver, everything looks great."

Basically, *Trust us, kid, and let us do our jobs.* He also challenges me to write out a detailed list of things I want to do when I get out of the hospital. This helps shift my thinking, and his advice about allowing myself to have bad days is freeing. So, I let myself be sad when I need to, but I give myself a time limit of one hour. The trick is not to dwell in Depression-Ville. Visit it, say hello, and get the hell out. That night, I type out a list in the Notes on my phone:

I will hug my friends and family.
I will go to Hawaii.
I will eat at Carmine's in NYC.
I will have Erica and others come visit.
I will see a Broadway show.
I will see nurse Dorothy's house.
I will get a dog and name her ECMO.
I will go to a movie.
I will sit by the fire at my mom's house.
I will write my next book of poetry.
I will work.
I will eat my mom's food.
I will eventually do gentle yoga.

It is reassuring to hear that the doctors are pleased with my progress, even if it doesn't feel like I'm making much. So, remember how the gastroenterologists did a colonoscopy plus endoscopy and couldn't find anything? Well, I'm bleeding again, so guess who gets to do everything all over? Yay!

As an added layer of frustration, I have four-hour dialysis sessions three days a week, which takes huge blocks of time. I am still trying to work with the physical therapist and speech therapist, which are hard to schedule around dialysis. On top of that, there are various procedures which, when adding in all the transport back and forth, can easily eat up a half a day. Still, I try to focus on the fact that my heart and liver are kicking ass. These are just "minor speedbumps," as Dr. MacArthur calls them, that are popping up.

One day, the TNT movie channel is showing the *Rocky* movies in order. I let myself watch and absorb them all, thinking and dreaming of what it would be like to be able to run up the famous steps in Philadelphia like Sylvester Stallone. Though I have never been a boxer, let alone attended a boxing match, I identify deeply with Rocky. A local fighter with zero professional boxing experience who is offered an incredible opportunity to go up against the heavyweight fighting champion, Rocky is a complete underdog and he knows it. The first time Rocky goes running, he is slow and stiff, barely making it up the steps before doubling over and gasping for air before slinking down the stairs. We watch his progression as he continues to train, until that triumphant moment when he bounds up the famous stairs again, this time like lightning, and we see his silhouette against a bright winter sky, arms raised in hard-earned victory. I am fighting my own kind of battle, and Rocky reminds me that the good only comes after the grueling.

*

The physical therapist, Ben, is the one to get me up and walking. He patiently helps me slowly slog to the side of the bed and shows me how to lift myself to standing—by leaning forward and using the legs—and then outfits me with a mask and walker. This is in tandem with a nurse who manages the IV pole and the respiratory therapist who manages the portable vent. It is somewhat of a production and takes at least fifteen minutes.

During my first attempt on January 10th, I make it to the outside of my hospital room door and back. The next attempt is to the drinking fountain right across the hall from my door. Baby steps, and certainly not far, but sometimes an inch can be more than just an inch. I grasp on to this glimmer of upward and forward mobility and try to fan it, like a flame.

Jake is not only a great nurse, but funny and personable. He often accompanies me and Ben on walks, out of necessity, and after seeing me watch the *Rocky* movies, starts playing music. He starts, of course, with "Eye of the Tiger" by Survivor. It becomes a bit of an anthem. I am working on regaining strength and balance, so I use a walker. In addition to a respiratory therapist manning the portable vent and a nurse on one side of me, someone follows with a chair so that I can sit down if I need. But Jake, ever the jokester and motivator, turns off the music if I sit down too soon. He is try-ing to get me to push myself, and rightly so. When he stops the music, I look at him, a bit exasperated, like, *Come on, man.*

"You gotta work for it," he encourages.

We listen to Lady Gaga, the *Hamilton* soundtrack—espe-cially "My Shot"—and Prince. Duh. By the 28th of January, I'm starting to make good strides. From my mother's journal on the 28th:

Up in chair 9:30? Walked to end of hall and around the corner with Ben. Did great. Advanced GI now saw endoscopy possible 29th or 30th. She is trying 5 over 5 pressure support [this refers to the trach] but needs reassurance to do it as she feels like she is taking lots of breaths. Ralph and I heard her speak even without valve on.

✳

So, what the whole "pressure support" thing means is this: the Respiratory Therapists can change the pressure support setting on the ventilator to allow the patient (moi) to attempt to breathe on their own, thus, how patients are eventually weaned off. The less support from the vent, the more the patient is breathing on their own. Right now, I am not having much suc-cess with breathing on my own very long.

But back to the current bleeding problem. Doctors want to do another colonoscopy and endoscopy to try to find the source of the bleeding. Fun times! My mother's journal from the next day, Wednesday, January 29th:

Dialysis started at 9am. Said GI procedure around 3pm. All teams in this morning. Finished dialysis with 2.5 liters. Rested then got in chair and then PT Ben came in and did some up-downs in chair then walked to hall window and back. Very confident and no sit down rests. Back in chair. Then GI said it would be 8pm and 4 patients in front of her. At 6pm lady

Advanced GI doctor, Dr. Sharaeh Moraveji came into room and told Aimee they still had 2-½ cases to go and she had her choice of being on schedule at 9:30am tomorrow or very late tonight. She chose tomorrow. Continues to be NPO.

Flashback to the night before: Dr. Moraveji had come in around ten o'clock the night before, extremely apologetic, her eyes betraying her tiredness and her mussed, curly hair peeking out from under her scrub hat. She said, "If you want, we will stay and do the procedure now, or we promise to get you in first thing in the morning."

Now, no matter how tired or hungry I am, I figure a tired and hungry doctor is worse, so I opted for the first thing the next morning. Plus, getting it out of the way first is always appealing. And the next morning, bright and early, I am rolled down.

As January rolls into February, the tests and therapies continue. More biopsies, more walking. One day, a different physical therapist comes in, very upbeat and positive. Let's call her Polly. As she talks, she tapes a huge, poster-sized piece of paper on the wall and begins to make notes. Notes like *"ten up-downs in a row,"* and *"use bedside commode, not bedpan,"* and a couple of other things that feel beyond my capabilities at the moment.

I look at my mom and she can see the absolute defeat wash across my face. I am nowhere near being able to get up and use the bathroom in time (suffering from continual diarrhea caused by the tube feeding), nor being able to do ten up-downs in a row. An up-down (in my case) is when you sit in a chair, place your hands on the armrests, and stand. Sounds simple, yes? Polly might as well have asked me to run a marathon. The mental and physical effort it takes to: A) get into the chair; and B) hoist myself up, is just not there yet. I physically squirm between feeling disappointed in myself and admitting the realities of the moment. My mom looks at Polly and says kindly, but realistically, "Aimee is not there yet."

Polly, remaining upbeat, acquiesces and says, "That's okay. Start smaller. How about three up-downs?"

I sigh in relief. After all, mountains are not climbed in a day, but instead made up of a thousand small steps. I start with three up-downs. But I still feel defeated. I try to remember Rocky. He started at the bottom, too, right?

✻

According to psychologist and professor Dr. Amrisha Vaish, negative bias is the capacity for adults to "attend to, learn from, and use negative information far more than positive information," according to an article in *Psychological Bulletin.*[11] It has been handed down over thousands of generations as a means to combat environmental threats—such as weather and predators—and served to act as an instinct for survival. Although society has outgrown worrying about the threat of predators, we still harbor the residue. We are still prone to shun things we view as negative. Like the potential of being rejected, going to the doctor, and, in my case, up-downs!

But, as clinical psychologist Dr. Madhuleena Roy Chowdhury points out, when we practice gratitude—and it is a practice—our brain "releases dopamine and serotonin, the two crucial neurotransmitters responsible for our emotions," according to an article called, "The Neuroscience of Gratitude and How It Affects Anxiety & Grief," on *PositivePsychology.com* in April 2019.[12] Every time we practice gratitude, we are strengthening those neuropathways and giving ourselves a mood boost in the process.

As anyone who has been through a mental and/or physical trauma can attest, there are always two sides to recovery: the physical recovery and the mental recovery. As hard as my physical limitations are at the moment—not being able to walk without help, being hooked up to a ventilator, not being able to get to the bathroom, enduring endless procedures ranging from daily blood draws to heart caths—those can, at least, be endured. Sometimes it is much harder to pull your psyche out of a dark place.

Lying fairly immobile in a hospital bed attached to IVs, monitors, and a ventilator is the absolute darkest place I have ever been. This feels like rock bottom. The good thing with being at the bottom is, as they say, there's only one way to go. So, I start practicing some daily gratitude:

I'm grateful for no procedures today. I'm grateful for no dialysis today. I'm grateful for Mom being here with me. I'm grateful for the kind nurses and Netflix. I'm grateful for my donor and their family. I'm grateful to be alive.

When facing your own mortality, it's natural to assess belief systems. I believe in reincarnation. I believe in miracles. After living this life, how could I not? I believe a man named Jesus lived and was crucified for his beliefs. I believe he advocated for the poor and the needy and would be one-hundred-percent against organized religion.

I believe a prayer recited aloud, alone in the woods, is as worthy as a prayer whispered in the mind in a church. I believe in the traditions and ceremonies of the East and the West. I believe in reflexology as well as vaccines.

I believe I was meant to be born with this imperfect heart just as much as I believe in the science that allowed surgeons to alter it.

I believe that in certain times, and under certain circumstances, the veil between the living and the dead is as thin as cellophane. I was always drawn to New York City and Paris, even before I had set foot in each one. There's a reason that I wanted to move to New York City the first day I was there, or that one of my happy places is a café in Paris called Le Select. (Though, I admit, who wouldn't be happy in Paris?)

I believe our physical bodies are an elaborate, temporary jumpsuit for our souls. Both are connected, but I believe that once our physical form has succumbed to the problem of being human, the soul is called to evaluate that particular lifetime's lessons and has some input on its future reincarnated form. And I have receipts for this.

Dr. Brian Weiss is a therapist-turned past-life regression expert who has appeared on *Oprah* multiple times and authored many books, including *Many Lives, Many Masters* and *Only Love Is Real.* He explains his belief that the universe is like a huge classroom. People are in all different grades, from kindergarten to doctorate programs. Each human lifetime is a chance to learn supremely spiritual lessons. He explains, in his many books, his view that upon death, the soul meets with a group of "Masters" for some self-evaluation. The soul and the Masters then map out a plan, or lessons to be learned in the next life. This happens over and over until a soul reaches a state of enlightenment. He says many times in his books that the main tenet of every major religion is love and I feel this to be true. He also talks a lot about attachment to people, to things, to situations. As he says in a post on X, formerly known as Twitter: "Happiness comes from within. It is not dependent on external things or on other people."

I can't begin to pretend to have a smidgen of the answers of the universe, but I know that love and gratitude are two keys. And in terms of my present situation, I am going to, as Dr. Weiss says, make my own happiness from within and tend to it like a garden and water it with the pleasures of small things. Watching *The Price is Right.* Days without procedures. The harp player who spends forty-five minutes outside my room on a challenging day.

"Happiness," says Weiss, "is rooted in simplicity."

I am hoping to eventually find some of that simplicity.

FIFTEEN

SUNDAY, FEBRUARY 2ND IS SUPERBOWL SUNDAY, SO OF course Mom and I watch the game, and according to my mom's journal, I "walked really well." The next day, Dad comes for a week-long visit from Palm Springs. Dad is great at many things, but, as he says, "Your mother is better at the medical stuff." It is a fun, good week, though medically complicated and tiring. I take my first walk, at Ben's gentle insistence, without the walker. He drapes two gowns around me, front and back, and guides my feet into my fuzzy slippers. I hold on to him for dear life as he supports me, his hands at my waist, and Dad follows with a chair.

"Look at you go," says Ben. This is the second short walk of the day; everyone has started pushing me to walk more. In the meantime, my dialysis catheter has become infected, so it needs replacing. I am also taken down for what feels like the umpteenth heart catheterization this week.

My dad spends a bit of time on the phone with my mom relaying what the doctors say and keeps her informed as best he can. This is not his comfort zone and, without Mom here, I feel a little unmoored myself. We take advantage of the nice weather and get outside. In fact, the doctors are insistent about this. So, myself (in a wheelchair), Dad, a nurse, and a respiratory therapist escape to the beautiful little courtyard to enjoy some sunshine, which feels like a warm gift to my sun-deprived skin. The temperature is in the high fifties, but is invigorating and the whole place oozes of tranquility and calmness. I try to soak it in like a sponge. I turn my face to the light and close my eyes for a minute.

While outside, we see and hear the hospital helicopter. It is the same helicopter the doctors used to procure my organs a couple of months ago.

"Isn't it amazing," my dad says in my direction as we gaze up, less about the helicopter and more about the unfathomable gift that we have been given.

✳

Mom returns on the 10th, just as I am working once again with the speech therapist and the Passy Muir valve. I have gotten better at it and can now use it for extended periods of time without feeling like I'm drowning.

"Say something to her," the speech therapist encourages.

"I'm glad you're back," I say, and we all laugh.

I am in pretty good spirits, but still bleeding, so I am given six units of blood over the next few days. Two seps forward, one step back.

On Valentine's Day, Brigitte, one of my nurses, gifts me a teddy bear, who I promptly name "MacArthur," and some other things. This act of genuine thoughtfulness, along with the ordeal of hospitalization, pops me like a balloon, and, just for a minute, I cry. Tears fall like tiny prayers, soaking into my gown.

I have always tried to be a grateful and gracious person, and I am overwhelmingly thankful for my second chance at life and my selfless donor, but there are still extremely challenging days. I know I will leave the hospital at some point; the end is not yet in sight. I also know that while there are many things I can't control, I can control my gratitude. I begin to start and end each day by mentally acknowledging two specific things I was grateful for, simple things, such as warm blankets and "Family Feud."

Remember the rollercoaster? I have developed an infection in the dialysis port lines, which is a concern, considering the lines run right to my heart. I will spare you the whole drama in getting the lines replaced, but just know that the opening line of my mom's journal for Wednesday, February 19th regarding the whole saga is: "CLUSTER FUCK DAY!" written in all caps and underlined three times. My mom's journal from Sunday, February 23rd:

Aimee started texting me at 1:30 am as she started having bloody stools — and they were going to give her blood. By the time I arrived at 10am she had had 3 units of blood and about 8 bloody stools. Tube feeds stopped. Bedside endoscopy done from 1:30-2:30. No sites found but all stomach and gut tissue is fragile and oozed when scope touched it. Back to the drawing board. She is puffy and fluid overload and can't do trach collar. Tried. MacArthur came in and told her to set goals for week/ outside/walk/trach collar. Kidney team in and fluid needs to be removed tomorrow.

Okay, so now it is time I tell you about February 25th, in which I blame technology for the failed endoscopy. The doctors and nurses prep me for another endoscopy. They are going to try a new tactic by inserting a camera in the shape of a small pill that will travel through my intestinal tract, helping them to find the exact source of the bleeding. One of my favorite nurses, Brigitte, makes it a point to be assigned as my nurse that day. I'm prepped and sedated without a hitch. It only feels like I've been out for less than a minute when I come to. As it turns out, the pill camera is not working, so the whole procedure is aborted! Because, of course, the camera isn't working. The Aimee Factor. So, they make plans to do this all over again.

The next day, I wake up completely unable to hear anything. For weeks, I have been asking if someone could clean out my ears; I know this is massive wax buildup. Mom calls the speech therapist, Sandra, since we figured my lack of hearing would impact her ability to work with me. Sure enough, she calls someone and later that afternoon, a wonderful pair of ENT nurses roll in a couple of interesting-looking contraptions. My mom looks at me, preempting any smidge of a resistant attitude and says, "Whatever they want to do, let them!"

First, they use a high-pressure water apparatus to apparently drown anything and everything in my ears, then a vacuum that sounds and feels like it is sucking out my soul from way below the earth. I can hear and feel large globs of yellow wax being extricated and I am overcome with relief and gratitude at being able to hear again.

✳

Saturday, March 7th marks my 45th birthday, and I cannot help but muse about what I might have done on this special birthday that happens to fall on a Saturday. Perhaps I would have had some friends and family gather at a local watering hole? Perhaps I would have hit Vegas with a bestie? But it is all moot, because this year, *life* is the ultimate gift. I am filled with love and warm fuzzies by all the sweet birthday messages on and off social media, and I am particularly jazzed that 80% of the messages invoked Prince or Paris, France, my two ultimate favorites. It is a happy, though busy, day. My mom's journal from that day:

45th birthday! Arrived back at 1pm with sheet cake for nurses in Aimee's honor. Dialysis day — she is puffy and feet dent when I push in. Asked kidney team to take off more fluid. Took 2½ liters. Dermatology here for leg rash. Petechiae (rash) from leg squeezers? Applied cream and said no to skin biopsy. Nurses came in and sang to her with Bday cake and card. Had walked to end of hall in the morning without stopping. Left at 7pm.

As Mom notes, Dr. MacArthur and the nephrology team have been working on getting the excess fluid retention under control. From a cardiac standpoint, MacArthur and team want as little excess fluid on me as possible, since that makes for better heart function. Dialysis helps with taking off the extra fluid, as well as doing the work of cleaning my blood in lieu of my non-functioning kidneys.

It is around this time that Dr. Chertow, the nephrologist whom we adore due to the dapper bow ties he always wears, talks to us about a probable need for a kidney transplant in the not-too-distant future. Normally, I might be crushed and incensed at having to think about another transplant surgery while recovering from one, but as you might be aware, dear reader, "normal" flew out the window eons ago.

"How long is the surgery?" I mouth to Dr. Chertow, with Mom translating.

"Two to three hours," he says. I ask how long I would be in the hospital afterwards.

"Five to seven days," he says.

"Sign me up!" I mouth, and make big check mark motion in the air, causing everyone to laugh. Compared to my current record of most consecutive days in a hospital ever, five days sounds like a vacation. Five days for a new kidney and no dialysis?! I'll take that tradeoff, please.

✳

Lest you think, dear reader, there isn't enough to worry about, I submit: The VAT Procedure Due To a Botched Paracentesis: A Short Story. I have, due to said botched paracentesis that happened around the 1st of December (pre-surgery), developed an infection in my gut. I have had at least half a dozen paracentesis procedures so far, but let's flashback to this particular paracentesis as the culprit. First of all, performing this procedure requires the doctor to insert the needle in just the right spot as determined by ultrasound. The trick is finding a spot where the abdominal wall is thin enough to extract the fluid, but not so thin as to puncture the gut. Since Stanford is a teaching hospital (which I fully support), on this particular day, a resident, not a doctor, is doing the procedure under guidance.

As the resident is extracting fluid, I detect a tinge of pink in the normally yellow fluid. She has accidentally drawn blood. I'm not really alarmed, though I do notice, as do the resident and the observing doctor. No fluid is able to be extracted, so the resident tries a new spot, with success, though at a cost. The resident is beyond mortified and upset with herself for this screw up. Her eyes shine with tears and she apologizes over and over. I assure her I don't hold any grudges, and I don't. It is what it is. Things happen. If you're thinking, *What the hell?! I would be livid!* Sure, you might feel every right to be livid, and you wouldn't be wrong. I simply suggest to ask yourself: is being livid going to correct the situation? Probably not.

✳

But back to the current infection. It requires a procedure called VATS, a video-assisted thoracic surgery where surgeons go in and clean out the lung. Surgeons had done this on my right lung, with minimal post-procedure pain, though I had rocked two additional chest tubes for a few days. So how did this one leave me screaming for morphine? Let's see, shall we? My mom's journal entry for Monday, March 9th:

VATS procedure scheduled for am — waiting on that. Emergency pushed hr back. RT James trying to get a walk in now (11:30)... 2:30pm and still waiting on VATS! Came to take her just before 5pm. Waited till 10pm for her to return. Dr. Lui left a voice message that things went well. Her face is very swollen and they said that is because they had her head down and feet up during the procedure. Finally left around 1:20am. Leah came on as her nurse around 12am. Aimee is in extreme pain (10!) asked for morphine!

Mom is there when I am rolled back into my room post-procedure at one o'clock in the morning. I come out of anesthesia screaming and crying in agony. She can attest that I have absolutely never cried from physical pain in my life. A nurse asks me what my pain level is on a scale of one to ten and I thrust both of my hands and all my fingers out and mouth: TEN! My side feels like it has been devoured by a carnivorous beast and my now mangled entrails are on the outside. I mouth to my mom through sobs:

"Please get me morphine!"

I can only imagine how it felt to have to tell your daughter in agonizing pain that they cannot not give you what you are begging for. The pain is so blinding and unrelenting that I don't even open my eyes. My face is completely swollen and flush, because at some point in the procedure, they had me basically upside down. Eventually, I calm down and drift off to sleep. I give that VATS a 0 out of 10. Definitely do not recommend. Hard pass.

A song I have loved since its release in 1997 is called "Shatter" by Merideth Brooks, which contains a lyric about how even if she cracks, she will not shatter. It is a punk rock anthem of survival, of determination, of grit. For me, the line also contains an apt nugget of advice on resilience. It is a reminder that, as the saying goes in contemporary pop psychology, it's okay to not be okay. Of course, 1997 was many years before mental health was truly taken seriously by society. In this line, Brooks reminded me—as well as a generation of Gen X ladies smack dab in the middle of middle-age adulthood—to have a mini breakdown to assuage a major breakdown. She sings that she simply breathes in and breathes out. One breath at a time. Like letting the air leak out of a balloon slowly to keep it from blowing up in your face, Brooks' lyrics give me permission to let just a little steam (read: fear) off, so that I don't completely shatter.

Still, right now, there continue to be more tough days than not. My mom's journal entry from Thursday, March 12th:

Hard morning. Told me she is scared and afraid she will never leave the hospital. No bowel movements for two days. Now they want to do stool softener and laxatives. Pain at 1-2. Finished dialysis at 6pm. 3 liters removed. Dr. MacArthur came in to talk to her during dialysis and told her to think positive; don't get in her head so much and worry. Start dreaming about getting out of here! Make goals this Sunday for next week. Told her if she hasn't started trach collar by then, ok, but she can ask for it whenever she wants to try and take it slow. Must sit in a chair and walk. Told diarrhea is ok right now if it happens after laxatives. Just before I left she was having first bowel movement.

As Mom notes, this is a particularly hard day, for no other reason than the three months buildup of worry, anxiety, and the enormity of all we have thus far been through. I am worried that I will never leave the hospital. I am worried that I will lose my left leg to amputation, where I am still experiencing some slight neuropathy from the Impella pump. Okay, so no, I am never going to lose my leg, as the doctors reassure me, but my mind is just dogpiling on me at this point.

Recovery is not linear, as I am learning. It is a thorn-infested trail full of potholes that winds back around on itself. My usual medical *modus operandi* is to let others worry until I absolutely have to worry. But I am starting to worry about my (lack of) bowel movements and, more concerning, the on-again, off-again bleeding. The constipation is taken care of easily enough with some stool softeners and laxatives, but I am becoming particularly worried that I have made seemingly little to no progress of getting weaned off the ventilator.

I am still not able to breathe completely on my own,

which, you know, is kind of something they want you to be able to do before they discharge you. A combination of underdeveloped lungs since birth and massive surgery means my lungs are taking their sweet time recuperating.

Some days I have to force myself to look for the sliver of light amongst the muck. Some days the sliver is simply being alive enough to make it through a day and commit to tomorrow. And that must be enough. Like the saying goes, it's always darkest before the dawn. Sunlight only exists because of the night.

❋

As for events taking place outside the hospital, back to current world events and the brewing international shutdown the world is facing in the beginning months of 2020. My mom's journal entry on March 13th:

Walked in this morning as I arrived (late). Guards at doors for screening questions for the COVID 19 virus. All nurses on Aimee's floor were masked and one patient was perhaps contagious for something — then later in the day all masks were off — [Aimee] felt much better. One chest tube removed — decreased lidocaine drip. Kidney team in and she asked for a puff [additional dialysis treatment to remove excess fluid only] to remove more fluid — 2 liters. Hands better but feet still puffy. Stomach side left [chest tube] is still draining. Loose brown stool. Good day and she was happy and in a good mood. Did trach collar for 2 hours late in day.

One thing this journey has taught me is to take the small victories. Four hours of uninterrupted sleep? Victory! One of five chest tubes taken out? Victory! Walked fifty feet? Victory! As the saying goes, Rome wasn't built in a day, and if it had been, the foundation likely would have crumbled. Another thing that life, and this journey, have taught me over and over is that things never stay bad forever. And, also, things never stay good forever. Rather, life is a shifting sand between the two.

As you are aware, dear reader, by March of 2020 the world has been reeling with the COVID-19 pandemic for months. Things are getting dire and faint whisperings of visitor restrictions are starting to circulate. On March 15th, one of my favorite nurses, Adam, comes in bearing a single sheet of paper and approaches quietly, head cast down.

"I'm so sorry," he says, handing the sheet to my mom.

It's the hospital's new lockdown policy.

As of the next day, the hospital will be closed to visitors. That means Mom must leave and will not be let back in for at least two weeks. (Two weeks would prove to stretch to months.) This is a bit of an emotional blow, as I not only like having Mom there in the hospital with me, but she typically takes part in all big medical discussions and is superb when it comes to remembering what all the doctors say each day during rounds, which she, more often than not, makes a point to be around for. Mom has been dealing with my medical uniqueness since I was born, and I almost always defer to her judgment.

For decades, I had taken a backseat approach to my medical situations—I let the doctors do the tests, let them tell me what needs to be done, then let them do it. But this journey has made Mom even more of an advocate for me than she already has been and made me realize that I must take a more active role in my healthcare, as well as learn to advocate for myself. As my dad liked to joke, "They [doctors] are the coaches, but we are the quarterback." Now, I am losing my first stringer. And, yes, of course my family talks in football analogies.

Since neither of us have much time to grapple with this, we do the best we can to figure out some semblance of a plan. FaceTime in the morning and night. Texting anytime, night or day. Get her on FaceTime when the doctors come in.

Truth is, I am in the best possible place I could be as a

recent transplant patient during a pandemic. My mind knows this, but my compromised, weak physical body and post-trauma brain just want to have my mom close. Her presence is part of my, and maybe her, healing. In the Facebook group on March 16th, Mom writes:

Dearest Team Aimee!!!!

Boy, the world is in a tizzy, and as we all, collectively, take a deep breath, grab a pair of Depends and hunker down for the immediate future, I wanted to ask your help. The hospital is locked down to visitors (I was thinking I was almost an employee) and Aimee and I are texting and FaceTiming our medical meetings with doctors. As of last night, I had to say bye bye to my daughter.

Please continue to cheer her on from your bunker now more than ever. She has a few procedures coming up this week and she is one smart and capable woman that can do this on her own, just wish she didn't have to. She is well loved there at Stanford, and being able to have the luxury of FaceTime to discuss medical issues together with her doctors is so helpful.

The snow has been plentiful up at my house so I won't get to drive home until most likely Wednesday as my Prius does not like that stuff!!! Ralph and I can hunker down there and keep clear of crowds together. I will update as I can.

Please Please all of you lovely loving folks stay safe and well! Sending virtual social distancing hugs your way! XO 🖤

It is a truth that the only constant in life is change, and this is just another punch we have to roll with. So, she packs up her bags and, thankfully, manages to get out of town and back home to Camino a few hours away before curfews and travel restrictions go into effect.

Although I like to think of myself as a tough cookie, and for the most part I am, I have a hard time adjusting to not having anyone there, but especially my mom who has navigated and weathered this entire journey with me. She makes sure that we both understand what the doctors say and what is going on; she is a deft and skilled medical translator. But also, she is, and always has been, my emotional support pillow. Mom's Facebook post on April 4th:

Hi Team Aimee 🖤 Late here in CA on a Friday night. Took this pic months ago and now the joke's on me, and you!!! The update on Aimee is that she remains in Stanford ICU, slowly working her way off the support of the ventilator; still receiving dialysis minimum 3 times a week; the small bowel obstruction that had occurred almost 3 weeks ago seems to be resolving (fingers crossed).

As this pandemic scorches our globe 🌑 Aimee remains safe and working on her recovery daily when scheduling permits. We try to FaceTime almost daily and often she calls when doctors come in to discuss medical issues. Grateful beyond words for video calling!

Last Sunday we set up a Zoom video call with me, Johnny, Tiffany, 4 kids and Aimee's pup, and her Dad. We will try and do that again this week 😊. We hope it gives her cheer as it certainly helps all of us! I so look forward to the day when the trach is out and she can talk and eat again!!!!! I know you all join us in praying that all stay safe during this horrendous virus and we can once again be with Aimee as she continues her fight for recovery. No one I know has more guts than she does! 💪

Remain in your quarantine and do all that you need to stay safe. This year has changed us all in many ways, and I would like to think 'for the better' when all is said and done. Learning patience from Aimee is now paying off dividends for me. May we all walk this walk with Grace and a large dose of humor. No excuses now for a lack of Spring Cleaning!!!!

Sending you all Love and warm wishes. Stay home and safe! Cuddle your resident quarantined families and your critters.

Drop Aimee a funny or something thought provoking... if YOU are feeling isolated and a bit down, remember she has been in hospital and away and isolated from all she loves for 6 months and counting. We've got this

Hugs and Smiles from a safe distance 😊🤗💜

As she says, we start setting up weekly Zoom calls with her and Ralph, Dad, Johnny and his family. Though I mostly listen as they talk, it is good to see everyone and gives Mom a chance to fill them all in on my progress. And like she says, we are all grateful for video calling!

The rest of March and April flit away with tests, procedures, and dialysis; a general melancholy has settled in me like a dampness, a permanent, pervasive fog in the spirit. I don't remember many details, but some things do stand out, like the four weeks when I have an abdominal x-ray taken daily after they discover that small bowel obstruction that Mom mentioned above, most likely a culprit of being bed-ridden for so long.

I dread this daily x-ray to check on this obstruction. It requires me to be laid flat onto the hard metal x-ray plate that runs from my armpits to lower bum. Not only does it sometimes take two people to get me into position, but laying on the plate is also excruciatingly painful due to a bed sore I developed post-surgery around my sacrum from lying in bed 24/7 for months. Right on the tailbone, it is the size of a quarter—raw, inflamed, painful to the touch, and a constant source of physical soreness. Oh, did I not mention the bed sore before? Must have forgotten in all the fun.

Anyway, back to the x-rays. The hardest and most physically excruciating part is getting the metal plate situated under my lower back and abdomen. One method is to slide it underneath me, starting at my head and scooch it down my back—until it hits the wound, at which point I scream silently and usually cry; the pain makes me want to jump out of my skin. The other method is to have a nurse roll me to one side, have the x-ray tech place the metal plate down, then roll me back onto it. This was preferable, though it still caused massive pain and anxiety and required another person to help, which is not always available.

But trading thirty seconds of pain for being alive seemed more than fair, though each thirty seconds had me saying every curse word I could think of in my head at full volume. Crack so you don't shatter, right?

✳

Easter marks another holiday in the hospital. Although I'm not religious, I always enjoy the family time, the good food, and subscribe to what Jesus— the Middle Eastern Jewish version— stood for. And Easter represents the miracle of rebirth and resurrection after a tragedy. Speaking of tragedy, here's my view: get it all in at one time. April 15th, Easter Sunday, my sister-in-law Tiffany posts in the Facebook group:

Just as The Bunny was finishing up her duties early Easter morning, Aimee's sweet 15-year-old Elphaba returned to the Ether. Her sweet chihuahua body was warm and clean, wrapped in a blue star blanket cocoon with her own tiny bunny by her side, good music on the radio~drowned in moonlight~her soul sure to return soon in some other energy or being ⋄ ⋄ Another tough and tenacious angel out there now, watching over our girl, sending her energy for continued healing and recovery ⋄

Here's a video from Elphaba's adventures during her final seven months, spending all her days nestled among her cousins, lounging in the sun, getting lots of baths, and celebrating all the holidays in style! It's sure to leave a smile on your face during these weird times💜 105 in doggy years, that's pretty impressive. Aimee was as loving and perfect a match as little Elph could have ever imagined. Proud of them both, now and always 💜🐾 💜 Keep DEFYING GRAVITY, Aimee! All the hands and paws are lifted up to you and your health!

I am forever grateful that Elphie spent her last months being loved on by my nephew and nieces and family. I hope our departed family dogs Dusty, Scruffy, Bella, Blue, and Babe, greeted her on the rainbow bridge with happy tail wags and yips of hello. But, yeah, life can be a bitch.

SIXTEEN

SPEAKING OF THAT MINX ANXIETY, IT MAY OR MAY NOT surprise you, dear reader, that after months of being in the hospital and it now being closed to visitors due to COVID, I finally slip into a depression. Or, perhaps it is more noticeable now? I mean, duh? I had previously talked to a psychologist—post-surgery—but didn't feel that I needed help.

I was fully aware of being in the middle of a miserable quagmire. I had even had many visits from the social worker, whom I'll just call "H." H was sweet, younger than I (mid to late twenties) and perhaps didn't know what do with me. She was always deeply serious, almost to the point where I felt like she was attending my living wake whenever she visited. I admit to having a bit of resistance to her visits in a *don't bring your negative vibes around me* kind of way. However, post-lockdown, negative vibes sneak in and Mom stages a one-woman, gentle intervention over FaceTime.

"Aimee, of course you are depressed. Talk to the doctor and let them give you something," she mothered as mothers do. Obviously, she was right.

Lexapro to the rescue. I start on Lexapro around the beginning of April. On May 1st, I post this in the private Facebook group:

Hello All 🖤 *please forgive my MIA status. Just know that I feel and appreciate deeply the love and support from this group. I do see every post, and I thank you. You have really been a ray of light through a rough time. Forgive me if I have not interacted much, but recovery is mentally and physically exhausting. Still in the hospital BUT GOOD THING is that I am miles from where I was 2 months ago, and I think my mental mojo has finally kicked in to get past these last couple hurdles. I am hopeful that things will move a little quicker from here on out.*

Again, love to all and I will keep you posted!

That newfound "mental mojo"? Yeah, that is 100% the Lexapro. And thank every goddess in the universe for it. I have never been on any mood medication before, but when it works, it works. If there is something that can help get you safely to the other side of the dark, miserable swamps that you are guaranteed to stumble into during life, take it. Eighties kids will understand: what if Artax and Atreyu had been armed with Lexapro in the Swamp of Sadness?!

If you can hang on, the sands will shift. On May 15th, Mom posts in the Facebook group:

Some lovely, wonderful news to share this Friday night!!!! Aimee was moved out of ICU late today and up one floor to J5, a cardiac and transplant regular recovery floor!!! (She has been on the 4th floor ICU since January 6th)!!! Big step and big boost as she moves ahead. The weaning off the ventilator continues and she has been making good strides. Swallow tests coming up to see how soon she can take fluids and food by mouth. When she called today and yesterday, she had the speaking "valve in" and I loved hearing her voice!!! Wonderful balm for my heart.

Have a sunny smiling weekend!

This is a first big step forward–getting out of the ICU. Big jump forward, small shuffle back, as May continues on with a few more spontaneous bouts of bleeding. The GI team continues to be thorough and, besides finding one spot the team took care of weeks ago, they still can't account for why it continues happening off and on. This is frustrating, to say the least, but after Dr. MacArthur tells us that long-term use of a ventilator can cause that to happen, I can relax, because that, at least, is a reason that makes sense.

I continue walking, though I have started asking (well, miming) to wear a diaper on walks for a couple reasons. One is gravity. When you spend 97% of the day in bed not moving around, the minute you do get up and move around, your bowels say, "Oh, hey, ok, we're awake!" And since I have no bowel control at the moment, sometimes it only takes a few steps before I feel the need to go number two. Sometimes, I'll be halfway down the hall.

So, after one unfortunate and embarrassing instance of leaving a tiny brown trail down the hall, like a line of tiny ants, I am not too proud to ask for diapers. The other reason is that the feeding tube formula is notorious for going right through you, like a sad Mexican food substitute that you can't even taste. Again, trying to work with and embrace the predicably unpredictable.

Speaking of food, during the past few months of not being able to eat, I have become obsessed with Food Network cooking shows like "Guy's Grocery Games" and "Beat Bobby Flay" and "Cupcake Wars." This is particularly hilarious to my mom, as it is a standing family joke that I do not cook. Like, almost ever. For decades, I have been relegated to "booze and French bread" type assignments for family gatherings. I don't mind this; I know my lane.

There are two major reasons for this new obsession with food shows. One: I have been a fan of competition shows and game shows since Bob Barker. Heck, I've been raised around competition—it's exciting. Two: I have not had a bite of food since before surgery. Cooking shows are a way for me to eat vicariously, delighting in the chef's absolutely mouth-watering, inventive creations. I love watching the process. A jazzed-up shrimp scampi, a decked-out mushroom and Swiss burger oozing with cheese, a berry cobbler with homemade vanilla/mango ice cream. And a whole show dedicated to making the most delicious and wild cupcakes imaginable? I mean, what's not to like?

"Why are you doing this to yourself?" Mom asks, laughing at me. Because if I can't eat good food, at least I can look at it! More than a few times over the past few months, I have begged and pleaded through tears with Dr. MacArthur for a single cheeseburger. Apologetically, he shakes his every time, both of us knowing I cannot yet have solid foods.

"I will buy you your first cheeseburger when you get out of here," he always says.

Why could I not eat? The short version is because of the trach. There is a path to being able to eat with the trach; the first step involves working with a speech therapist and doing a swallow test to make sure you can still swallow properly. The first step of the swallow test involves a camera being inserted through the nose and down into the throat area so she can see if I am in danger of aspirating any food into my lungs. Having a camera threaded down through my nose is beyond a doubt the worst part of the whole process. Think about trying to take a thin straw and shoving it up your nose so far that it goes down your throat. It makes me gag.

The next step involves ingesting just the tiniest bite of applesauce doctored up with barium, which turns the applesauce the color of an overripe blueberry. It glows brightly on the x-ray, like slow lightning as it goes down. If I don't aspirate and the applesauce goes down the right way, I can start thinking of being able to eat.

But, dear reader, I fail the swallow test a second time, and I am still no closer to any cheeseburgers.

The only consolation is that, after this second failed test and much conversation, my team of doctors suggests putting the feeding tube in my abdomen—a common thing for long-term feed tube use. This would free me from the feeding tube in my nose, which has come out multiple times, despite best efforts to keep it in place. One time, it just fell out, like a thread being pulled, when I stood up. I cried bitterly at the reinsertion that had to happen. Inserting a feeding tube in the nose is not a simple process, nor is it pleasant. Imagine a thin, plastic tube shoved up your nose and making its way down the back of your throat into the stomach to reside right at the start of the small intestine. The inserting of the tube always makes me gag, and it makes my nose incredibly raw and sore.

After a short procedure (I mean, what's one more at this point?), I now have a new tube snaking out of my abdomen, and I'm thrilled to be rid of the dangling nose nuisance. Note to self: Always take the small victories.

Besides cooking shows, another series that I like to watch is the "American Ninja Warrior" competition. Although these competitors train intensely for the show, they have normal lives outside of being a part-time ninja. They are schoolteachers, medical professionals, mothers, nurses, and gym owners. I love and cling to the idea that non-professional athletes (though, could you really call them "non-professionals" after training and competing?) can push the limits of their bodies with such phenomenal results. Flying through obstacles with dangerous, exhilarating names like "Shrinking Steps," "Corkscrew," "Warped Wall," and "The Dungeon," each person grabs my rapt attention as I'm internally rooting for each one, cheering for them to reach the top and slam their hands down on the buzzer. And when they fall out of an obstacle, I feel every ounce of their disappointment. Being a coach's kid on the receiving end of a few brutal defeats, I can empathize with their utter disappointment. But, as Dolly Parton sagely says, you can't have rainbows without the rain.

But first, there must be the rain. On May 31st, Mom posts in the Facebook group:

Hi Dear Aimee TEAM 😎

Time for an update and request. As was posted a couple of weeks ago, Aimee was moved out of ICU on May 15. But she was moved back to ICU on May 22. The reason was her lungs could not expel the CO2 nor could she get enough oxygen. Many procedures later and a switch in trach valve that was leaking, they have determined via blood cultures that she once again has an infection of Enterococcus and pneumonia. She had not been out of bed for a week, so she took some steps the last two days but it will take some time to get her strength back to where it was a couple of weeks ago.

She continues her every-other-day dialysis as kidney function has not returned. Believe me when I say she continues to do all she can to recover. But it has proven to be a long road and she knows she has months still in front of her. At some point in her future will be a move from the hospital to a facility that concentrates on ventilator weaning and physical rehabilitation that will take some months.

At present her two transplanted organs have shown 0 rejection! We hold good thoughts that will continue. Because of COVID19 we still can't visit her, which makes her days quite long. If you would like to drop her a note or card her mailing address is: [redacted] A little encouragement from her Pals could go a long way right now 😊

Our family continues our weekly zoom visits, and Aimee and I (with docs and nurses) FaceTime nearly daily. We are all hanging in there and hope you are as well in these most difficult days. As you go about your daily activities and put a mask on for your safety and others think about Aimee... she is one of the ones most vulnerable. It makes the inconvenience personal and relatable. Much love from all of us to all of you 🖤😎😎

Yes, after a week of being on the fifth floor, as Mom mentions, I am moved back down to the ICU. After pushing myself to wear the trach collar (i.e., trying to breathe on my own), it is determined through blood tests that my lungs are still not expelling carbon dioxide from my body fast enough on their own, nor am I getting enough oxygen on my own. Basically, I have still not made hardly any progress on getting off the ventilator. Not to mention that too much carbon dioxide in the blood turns it more acidic and can cause a fun array of side effects, such as dizziness, fatigue, severe oxygen depletion, and, in the worst cases, death. This is what precipitates the move. I remember Dr. MacArthur visiting me on the fifth floor during the first day or two and he encourages me to wear the collar as much as I can. The next thing I really remember is being back in the ICU. I had grown extremely sleepy and lethargic due to too much CO2 in my blood and not enough oxygen, and my blood was super acidic. Whoops. So, back on the vent 24/7.

✳

As another month moves forward on the calendar and the weather continues to warm, Dr. MacArthur and others suggest getting me transferred to a rehab hospital. The truth is that despite the whole feeding tube, ventilator, and dialysis thing, I am lightyears ahead of where I was in January, post-transplant. There are, however, lightyears still to go. And, while Stanford is a world-class hospital, they are not in the business of rehab, which is what I now need.

On June 18th, I am transferred to a facility located a little over an hour's drive away. In everyone's opinion, this is a good move. We are told that this place specializes in weaning patients off ventilators, which is the biggest hurdle to springing me from medical captivity. My mom is allowed into the hospital on the day I am to be transferred, a gesture for which we are both extremely grateful.

Preparations go as smoothly as they can. My mom helps pack my backpack and one other small bag. She then loads all the other items that have accumulated over months into the back of her Prius. She arms me with a little notebook and pencil, so that I can "talk" to the medics if I need to, and I mouth my mother a request for a diaper for the drive, still not trusting my bowels. I am loaded onto the skinny, bumpy gurney with a little extra padding under the butt. The ventilator is prepped for transportation. While I still have IV ports for medications (since I cannot yet swallow pills), I am rarely hooked up to an IV, and the feeding tube is paused for the duration of the drive. This is our version of a "simple" transfer.

As I'm rolled to the elevators by one of my favorite nurses, M, and the medics, all of the nurses and aids on the floor have gathered to see me off, cheering and clapping. There is a huge, computer-printed banner that says, "Good Luck, Aimee!" that has been signed by everyone, which they later give to my mom. It renders me speechless and is truly touching. Mom gets the whole thing on video, and we take some pictures.

"I've never seen anything like that," one of the medics says mostly to the other medic when we are all alone in the elevator. "That's really something."

I smile, sending silent hugs and eternal gratitude to everyone at Stanford.

The journey is uneventful. Until, immediately upon arriving, I feel a familiar sensation and sigh in defeat. I have just bled in my diaper. A lot. As I am being unloaded from the ambulance, I quickly scribble a note and hand it to one of the very understanding medics.

"Okay," she says. "Don't worry. We got you."

The medics and Kentfield staff quickly do intake and get me into a room. The Kentfield nurses seem dismayed and put off by my accident. Still, they get me cleaned up and settled. My father has been in the loop on the transfer, and we have, somehow, gotten permission for him to visit for an hour that day. He arrives in the doorway with a big smile, despite, I'm sure, feeling out of place. He chats up anyone and everyone who comes in the room, taking notes of the names of doctors and nurses. "And what do you do?" is his standard follow-up question after asking and jotting down the person's name. Always a proponent of gathering information, my father is diligent in taking notes, phone numbers, and business cards from anyone who comes in the room during the ninety minutes (*shhh*) he is there. This is a trait I have, as of late, tried to cultivate. He has always had a "look before you leap and then look again" mentality, whereas I tend to use a looser "leap and figure it out on the way down" method. Interestingly, this journey is teaching both of us the value of these opposing mentalities. While he is having to work with a situation which he has almost no control over (which, I cannot overstate, is not his comfort zone), I am having to face and plan for the short and long term in a more practical and strategic way than I did in my old, bohemian, *laissez-faire*, "I'll figure it out" method.

Throughout that first afternoon, I am greeted and examined by the intake doctor, who gets my tube feed and medications ordered and administered. A dialysis nurse stops by, confirming he will see me tomorrow for treatment and that he has already spoken to the physical therapist to make sure there are no schedule conflicts. Although the facility is older and the rooms smaller than half the size of those at Stanford, to find the staff's proactiveness at Kentfield similar to Stanford is a comfort. But, as is typical, it takes a couple days for the bloom to come off the rose.

I will, dear reader, skip over the details of the next four weeks at Kentfield, and instead, stick to the highs and lows:

Low: for the duration, there are two patients' rooms guarded 24/7 with armed guards. I see the guards every day I walk and can't help wondering about the patients they are guarding; not about their dangerousness, but about their physical and mental state. In my worst moments, I imagine one of them breaking out of the room and going on a rampage down the halls.

High: by the end of the four weeks, I am able to confidently use the Passy Muir speaking valve and have daily conversations with Mom over FaceTime. I have also been working on the delegated swallow exercises and finally pass a swallow test for the first time. This is major! I am slowly allowed to eat pudding and puréed food. In terms of food choices, there are none, but I do not care. Bland and dry meatloaf goes down like prime filet and the chocolate pudding cup tastes like Italian gelato, as far as I'm concerned.

Low: I am still making little to no progress weaning off the vent. One day, the occupational therapist says, "Well, let's start working towards getting you ready to live with a ventilator at home." She wants to teach me how to get dressed and navigate daily life while on a ventilator. I shake my head and obstinately refuse. Being on a ventilator outside of a hospital is not an option. Period. That, universe, is pushing me too far.

High: I am able to make a full loop around the halls and, by the end, my general stamina is very much improved. The physical therapist is kind and patient with me, though he still makes me wear a belt around my waist when we walk for him to hold on to. Annoying, but policy. One day he challenges me to use just a cane, the kind with four prongs on the end. Reluctant at first, I wobble down the hall as he keeps me steady. This is good progress.

Low: I prop my phone six inches from my face to watch *Hamilton* the day it drops.

High: I watch *Hamilton* the day it drops and it is a revelation.

Low: We find out that insurance will only cover four weeks at a rehab facility, and my caseworker's job answers to dollars, so after weeks, I am sent back to Stanford, even though I am still not any closer to getting rid of the ventilator. As I am being wheeled into the elevator on my way out, my caseworker floats by. She barely glances my way while throwing a lazy and haphazard "good luck" toward me without breaking stride. It takes all of my will power to refrain from giving her the double bird.

High: On July 16th, I am transferred back to Stanford and Dr. Vagelos is on duty that night. Thank everything that is good and holy.

SEVENTEEN

I AM BACK AT STANFORD AND SETTLED IN SHORTLY after 8:00 PM. I immediately scribble a note to Dr. Vagelos asking if I can order some food. Typically, I am sure any doctor would want and need to clear this per their own hospital's guidelines and speech therapists, but Dr. Vagelos and I have a deep patient/doctor history. After relaying that I have passed a swallow test and have been eating puréed food and pudding for days at Kentfield, he lets me order food, God bless him.

Unlike Kentfield, Stanford has an abundance of good choices on the menu and, though I am still restricted to puréed foods and liquids, I don't care. It's real food. I order puréed macaroni and cheese along with a tomato bisque. I cautiously chow down while watching "Holey Moley," the comical putt-putt on steroids game show. The macaroni and cheese are like a yummy, light pasta and cheese souffle. The hot soup goes down warm and silky. Even the cranberry juice tastes like fine wine.

Except for the damn trach and dialysis, I am doing extremely well. Throughout all the biopsies, and other unrelated "medical potholes" as we liked to call them, my new organs are doing fantastic. This continues to help me and others stay positive. As long as the organs are working, the other stuff can be taken care of, just perhaps not as quickly as I would like.

Back at Stanford, a respiratory therapist named Henry, whom I met for the first time, starts working with me. We immediately begin working diligently for what feels like the millionth time on getting me off the ventilator, which is the only outcome I will accept. He studies my reactions as he tries different pressure-support settings, testing how far he can push me in getting me to breathe on my own before I need the support of the ventilator. And although I try to hide it, he can always tell when I still need support, muttering "damn" under his breath. It's a very subtle shift; I never gasp for air, but he senses the ever-so-slight change in my demeanor and face when I am not getting adequate oxygen.

A couple of days after returning to Stanford, the speech therapists want to do another swallow test to confirm that it is safe for me to be eating. A little frustrating, but I understand the protocol and reasoning. So, out comes the barium-laden applesauce once again.

Dear, reader, I fail.

I mean, I've had a few crying fits over the past months, but this hits me hard. I burst into tears and cry bitterly at the thought of not being able to eat real food again. Of course, it is temporary, but this colossal loss feels like an anchor around my spirit. I grieve my puréed macaroni and cheese, the puréed pizza, the puréed meatloaf. The speech therapist is exceedingly empathetic and offers to evaluate me again in a few days. Through snot-riddled sobs, I agree.

So, why the change? Was I not supposed to be eating the past week? Not necessarily; Stanford just has slightly stricter standards than Kentfield. It is noted that this test went a lot better than my previous test at Stanford months ago, but it's just not quite as good as they would like.

And, just like that, good things can happen. Stanford has, by this time, relaxed visitation policies, allowing one visitor per day, so my mom is able to visit, and it's the first time I've seen her in person in a month. She posts to the private Facebook group on Sunday, July 18th:

Let it be known that on this Saturday around High Noon, Aimee left her walker at the door and flew solo around the unit. It has been a great visit for Thurs, Fri, and today.

No telling what she will do by the next time I come down the mountain to see her. She has her own great game plan on weaning from the vent and getting on trach collar again, which then means eating a little again. Aimee looks good, feeling spunky, and doing whatever she can to move forward. She is a real Warrior Woman and definitely taking charge more!

I have gotten strong enough to walk the halls without a walker, which feels like a huge step forward, pun intended. Project "Get The Eff Out Of Here!" is starting to gain momentum. After languishing for months in a recovery stupor, seeing some concrete, tangible evidence that I am slowly getting my life back is a huge morale boost.

Towards the end of July, my dad comes to visit again. We take trips to the garden to enjoy the beautiful Palo Alto weather, sending frequent updates to Mom. On July 26th, she posts in the Facebook group:

Hope this brings a big smile to all your faces. Aimee's father has been visiting her the last 3 days and they just sent these great pictures of her outside on the deck at Stanford! Such a treat to see this. As you can see from the pics, she still is attached to ventilator support, but they are reducing it slowly every other day. Then they will start letting her breathe off the ventilator for short periods and work her way up. Her lungs and diaphragm have atrophied over these last many months, so it is a slow steady course of getting back her strength for her body to do it on its own. But she is trying! She is a magnificent Warrior and I remain in awe!

One particular image from this visit cracks me up. I'm standing outside dressed in two hospital gowns—one open (but tied in the back) and one worn like a jacket so that both my front and back are covered. I sport my fuzzy, brown LL Bean slippers gifted from my Aunt Shari a few years ago for Christmas and strike a supremely awkward disco pose as the ventilator tube snakes from my throat, down my body, then off to the left until it is lost to the frame of the picture. Laughter, as they say, is great medicine.

The next week, Mom returns and we venture out to the gardens again where the nurse decides to have a dance party. She pulls up Spotify on her phone and hands it to me. When you hand me your phone on Spotify, I'm going to play Prince. My mom's post to the Facebook group on July 31st:

A little Sunshine, a little 'Prince' music to dance to, the great help of Irene her nurse and Don her Respiratory Therapist, and Mom to hold camera and help navigate, well that makes for a win-win for all. So far her ventilator weaning is going slow and steady and she wants it gone in the worst way☺.

She says she has been dreaming of food every night, but then again I came in yesterday and she's hooked on watching the Food Network!!! HELLO! I can say that the difference I see from my last visit 2 weeks ago is huge! She is stronger and a lean mean fighting machine.

We hope your weekend brings blue skies, sunshine, and happy smiles your way (even if the only smiles you see are in the mirror!) Hugs and stuff from the 'A' Team 😄

A video from this visit shows me bopping along to "Let's Go Crazy" by Prince. Behind the mask, I can tell I am starting to piece together happy. Movement. Music. Sunlight. All of it medicine. And, as Mom relates, there has been noticeable forward progress over the past weeks.

And then, dear, reader, it happens. On August 5th, I post the following in the Facebook group:

And the speech therapist said, let unto her be brought tomato bisque and mac and cheese! She rejoiced, and so it was brought and it was glorious. Amen.

I have been cleared to eat again, starting with the purée diet again. Though I am not weaned completely off of tube feed (and won't be for another five months), I am elated. Another step closer in Project "Get The Eff Out Of Here!" My mom's post to the Facebook group on August 6th:

See this beautiful face? She is the BEST! See the little purple circle on her neck? That is called a Passy Muir valve and when she has that put on, she can talk and is now allowed to eat some foods!!!! She just called to say Hi as she was on the last half hour of kidney dialysis for today.

She is very encouraged as she now sees how close she is coming to being rid of the ventilator!!! And then the tracheotomy can be removed after that. Her lungs seem to be clear now and lung capacity and function as well as diaphragm are both improving after now 8 months post transplants and 10 months at Stanford (on Aug. 9th)! Does she have mountains yet to climb on this journey to a healthy discharge? YES, but she now has her hiking boots on and she is kicking butt! Let's all cross our fingers and push her to the next goal!

From here on out, it starts to get easier each day. Mom continues to visit and we watch the original *The Parent Trap* and *Hamilton.* Dialysis continues, as do daily walks, going further and getting a bit faster every time. I have now taken to stopping during my walks a couple of times to do some light stretching. I bemoan my lost yoga strength and flexibility after being so sedentary for so long. Still, I am grateful for wobbly, skinny chicken legs that somehow simultaneously weigh nothing and feel like lead, as well as the gentle soreness in my arms and back after doing some awkward sun salutations.

I also work on staying off the vent for large amounts of time. First step: breathing without the vent. Next step: walk around without the vent. On August 10th, I have the following text exchange with my friend Erica:

> **GUESS WHO JUST WALKED WITHOUT THE VENT TODAY**

> OH MY GOD ARE YOU SERIOUS?!!!!!

> THAT'S MY FUCKIN HOMEGIRL

And I post the following in the Facebook group:

So, yesterday I walked WITH my speaking valve in and NO VENT, just an oxygen tank. And today I walked TWICE with speaking valve and just oxygen tank. This is a HUGE step towards getting out of here and getting this lovely (ahem, sarcasm) trach out! I am super thrilled. I have been watching the Food Network, obsessing about good food, and my diet was upgraded a little today—so I'm off total purée diet. Life is grand.

This marks a true turning point. Never has the END seemed so close that I could reach out and grab it. A once-in-visible distant star, the end is now hurtling towards me, its bright light and warmth fueling me. Walking unassisted? CHECK. Eating? CHECK. Breathing on my own? ALMOST CHECK. Over the next week, I keep my speaking valve in more and more and rely on the vent less and less. I start posting a flurry of what my cousin dubs the "It's Happening People" posts in the Facebook group: On August 16th, I post:

PEOPLE, IT'S HAPPENING!

I was just moved up to the 7th floor, which is the last stop on the hospital merry-go-round! I was only on oxygen all day and night yesterday, so if I do that a few more days, I can say good riddance to my fashionable neckwear. YAY!!

This move to the seventh floor feels like surfacing after months of being under water. No more ICU. No more consistent monitoring. I am able to order whatever I want to eat, whenever I want. I get settled into the room and start negotiating with the nurse about wearing monitors. I agree to keep my oxygen cannula in my nose and the oxygen monitor on my finger, but ask for the heart monitor to be taken off, to which she agrees. All the IV medicines had recently been transitioned over to oral medicines, so I am now, as Southwest Airlines says, free to move about the cabin—and without a walker or cane!

I do, however, agree to let a nurse walk with me when I roam the halls. Unlike the hustle and sometimes frenetic energy of the fourth floor, the seventh floor feels like a clear and calm oasis of silence. Indeed, I feel, almost, like I am on vacation. Then, on August 19th, I post:

PEOPLE! IT'S STILL HAPPENING AND I AM NOT THROWING AWAY MY SHOT!

So, today they 'capped' the trach. Once I can tolerate this for 24 hours, I'M FREE! This will only take a day or two. Then they can take it out, toss it in the trash, and kiss it goodbye forever!

OH, and I'm in pajamas, as in, actual clothing!

Though I might be getting out of the hospital, there is still work to be done. I will need to put on some weight, build up my strength, and keep up with dialysis for a while, but I'm sure I can do that. Again, I would never have gotten through the past ten months without your support! It's strange when I think back to days that were so bad that I really didn't think I would make it out of the hospital. So I asked and raged at the universe for help and to just fix it.

The universe answered, but not in the ways I expected. A few months ago walked in Henry, a respiratory therapist, who really started turning things around. And Ben the physical therapist that put up with my absolutely cranky self and helped (made) me start walking. And so many other fabulous nurses and doctors.

It was the universe's way of getting through my thick skull that people are the change-makers. Prayers must be paired with action to come to fruition. Damn, and I thought I just needed a magic wand. Lol MORE SOON! 🖤

Moving to the seventh floor feels like a rebirth, the calming of a sea after hurricane. "Capping the trach" means just that. The long tube stretching from my neck to the ventilator is removed, while a black cap is placed over the trach site at the neck, meaning I am breathing 100% on my own. Procedure dictates that I must be able to breathe completely on my own without any support for at least 24 hours before the doctors will consent to removing the trach. This is what I had been working towards for months. Until now, I had only lasted a few hours without support before I needed to be put back on the ventilator. Slowly, my lungs have become strong enough to last a full day of breathing on my own.

The next day, August 20th, is the day. The removal of the trach is equally exhilarating and anticlimactic. It had lived in my throat for so long, I imagined it had become fused to my body somehow, but after the snipping of a few sutures, the tube—three-quarter inches wide and seven inches long— slides out easily. It is bigger and longer than I had imagined, but feels miniscule compared to the job it had done in keeping me alive for months. I have the nurses take pictures of me post-removal and immediately post it to Facebook:

PEOPLE!! LOOK!!!

THE TRACH IS OUT!!! (See that blue tube in the lower left corner... that's what was in my throat for months!) HALLELUJAH AND AMEN!

Swarmed with good wishes and congratulations, I start preparing for a day that I had sometimes thought would never come. Now that I can breathe on my own, I can be cleared to leave. Nurses make me do the requisite walks in the hall to "test out" my breathing post-trach removal, as per rules, but all goes well. I start bugging my mom about coming to get me and otherwise spend the day watching TV and eating. God, I can eat again! I pick up the hospital phone, call down to the kitchen, and, with my still slightly squeaky voice, order omelets for breakfast and raviolis for dinner. I take a shower. I watch movies and FaceTime.

Mom posts to the Facebook group on August 24th:

Hi, All you Glittery Unicorns!!

I hope this video brings you great Joy and perhaps a misty eye for helping to get Aimee to this amazing point. Discharge will happen in the next day or so, to travel up to live with Ralph and I and our herd of deer!

Had lessons today on how to hook up and run the feeding tube for 18 hrs a day to fatten up this skinny mini! Her taste buds haven't been affording her much appetite and she needs to eat to get rid of the lifeline to the feeding tube!!

I am incredibly excited for Aimee to get home, relax, move around the house, and regain her strength and stamina! Dialysis has been set up for MWF down the road from us in Cameron Park and then in a year or so she is planning to sign up for a possible kidney transplant! (Did I just day that? Yep, she is going for the trifecta!)

We love you all and are so grateful for sending Aimee your healing prayers and life force energy!

I pack my remaining belongings into a backpack, a carry-on suitcase, and a couple of hospital-issued brown bags. I pack my speaking valves from the trach to take with me. I pack any open packages of body wipes, tissues, etc. Computer, cords, slippers, robe, clothes, etc. When Mom had visited previously in June, she had taken home a trunk-full of gifts and "winter clothes" that had accumulated, but I had kept the small teddy bear gifted by one of the nurses, Bridgitte, named "MacArthur Bear" after my heart transplant surgeon. We had even put a mask on him when the world when into COVID lockdowns.

I put on my "Defy Gravity" t-shirt from the Broadway musical *Wicked* and make a video (with Mom's help) to post. I'm not literally defying gravity, but I do feel as if I have defied death a few times.

Dr. Lui comes by. Even though he wears a mask, I can tell by his eyes that he is grinning just as wide as I am. It's hard not to form a close emotional bond with doctors who have, more than once, saved your life. Mom and I both get a little teary-eyed as we hug Dr. Lui goodbye.

Dr. MacArthur, whom I had nicknamed "Hotty MacSurgeon," comes by. We are both ecstatic about my discharge. We take a selfie, though he keeps his mask on (because COVID) while I grin maskless like a maniac.

Before discharge, there is a whole checklist to take care of: meeting with the post-transplant coordinator, meeting with the pharmacist to go over the nineteen medications, learning how to use the food pump (more on that in a minute), having the last IVs removed, and, of course, meeting with the doctors on call. During this day and a half, my room feels like Grand Central. The coordinator asks me what I'm going to do when I get home. She means medically.

"Take my medications and go to clinic visits," I say immediately.

"Good girl," she says. You'd be amazed at the number of patients who don't bother to show up for clinic visits. Meds, on the other hand, are a life-long, non-negotiable. The immunosuppressants must be taken approximately twelve hours apart until the day you die. By artificially suppressing the immune system, they keep the body from attacking the new organs. As great as these medications are at keeping patients alive, they can come with side-effects and have not advanced much in thirty years. While billions of dollars are spent on R&D every year on technical medical advancements, which have led to tens of thousands of lives saved, more research is needed to improve the immunosuppressive drugs that patients must take for the rest of their lives.

Okay, stepping off the soap box. Though the trach has been removed and I can eat, I still need interim supplemental nutrition and I will go home with the feeding tube still snugly stitched to and hanging from my abdomen. This feels like an extremely small pittance to pay for being able to escape the hospital after so long. The technician shows us how to load the bagged food and work the machine that I will be attached to for at least eight to ten hours a day. It's light and attached to a pole that can be wheeled around. Like I said, this is a price I am more than willing to pay to go home. Finally, on August 25th, eleven months to the day of being admitted to Dell Children's hospital in Austin, Texas, Mom posts:

Eleven months ago today on Sept 25th, 2019, Aimee was admitted to the hospital in Austin TX! Today she will soon roll out of Stanford Hospital with a beautiful new heart ♥ and liver. So grateful to the donor and their family!!! The car ride will be the scariest thing she has done in almost a year!! Wish us luck 🙏🙌

I am masked up (because I received a transplant during COVID) and wheeled (because protocol) down the hall and into the elevator for the last time. Mom has pulled the car to the front and I practically dive in. It's about a four-hour car ride home, some of which I spend nodding off. In some ways, it is both the longest and shortest car ride of both of our lives, including the summer treks from Illinois or Texas to North Carolina.

We make it home around dinner time and I have never been so glad to sit at my mother's kitchen table than I am right now. Ralph unpacks the car, while Mom quickly whips up a batch of frozen ravioli for the three of us.

I sit at her kitchen table and savor it. It is the best ravioli of my life.

EIGHTEEN

EXCEPT FOR BEING READMITTED A WEEK LATER FOR five days due to minor issues and being sent home with an oxygen tank for the time being, things continue to improve. Since I am 88 pounds with clothes on at discharge, the feeding tube is still a temporary necessity. The day after we get home, we receive a large shipment of tube feed supplies. The food comes in pouches that we hang on the pole and then attach to the feeding tube. I am attached to the tube feed for ten to twelve hours a day and opt to have it attached from about nine at night to ten or so in the morning, so as to have as many "unrestricted" day hours as possible. We fill the outside fridge with Ensure, and I try to drink one every day. I order my favorite Cliff bars for dialysis snacks.

I am set up with dialysis at the closest clinic that is twenty miles away, three times a week, from 9:00 AM to around 1:00 PM on Mondays, Wednesdays, and Fridays. This will be pretty much the extent of my medical and personal obligations and outings for about a year. COVID plus transplant equals uber cautiousness. One of the nurses at the dialysis clinic, Laurie, introduces me to another patient, Madison. Soon, Madison and I start meeting up for lunch once a month. It's a chance for us both to get out of the house and do something fun.

On my first official clinic visit back a month after discharge, the coordinator, Kathy, asks how many doses of medication I missed.

I blink.

"None," I say. Mom and I have both been vigilant about this.

"Excellent!"

I start walking laps around the house and eating. I eat a lot. One of the medications is an appetite stimulant and it seems to be working, though Mom's amazing cooking is hard to resist anyway. My body is still adjusting to all the medications and, every once in a while, they trigger my upchuck reflex. This is temporary, though, and subsides.

Dad visits a couple times in the fall. For the most part, we sit on the couch and watch football.

My first social outing is in late October to a local winery for their pizza day. Still at the height of COVID, it is outside and I join a very small group of about seven people. Although I have no taste for wine, the pizza is phenomenal and I enjoy a good two hours outside during this lovely fall afternoon. Upon returning home, I promptly take a two-hour nap. Baby steps.

During this next year, I am also evaluated for and put on the kidney transplant list under a program at Stanford that allows liver transplant patients (hand raised) to move toward the top of the kidney transplant list if you get listed for a kidney within a year after your liver transplant. So, on December 8th, with days left to spare, we travel down to Stanford and meet with all the appropriate people. I am accepted to be a future transplant patient, and listed, but not yet activated. They still want me to beef up and continue to improve. We are going for the "transplant trifecta," as we like to call it. Plus, now that I'm listed, there's no rush to find a kidney, since people can, and do, survive on dialysis for many years, though that is not optimal.

Speaking of transplants, you might be wondering about my heart and liver donor. A year after transplant, recipients are allowed to write their donor's family through the UNOS network. In February 2021, I send a letter off to my coordinator at Stanford, who passes it on to UNOS, who gets it to the donor's family. I admit that I struggled to know what to say. I mean, what do you say to a grieving family who has lost someone, but, at the same time, saved your life? "Thank you" doesn't feel or come close to adequate.

But, say thank you I do. I tell them how grateful I am and assure them I will always do everything in my power to take the best care of their loved one's heart and liver. I tell them a little bit about me and ask to hear a bit about my donor.

Months and months pass. I am sitting in the dialysis chair when I get an email that I have a secure letter in my Stanford online portal. It's from the donor's mother, whom I'll call "J." I forward the letter to Mom, who is just as ecstatic to hear from the family. To keep my donor anonymous, I'll call her "K." K's mom describes her as a bright, beautiful thirty-two-year-old working girl who succumbed to a sudden cerebral aneurysm. Basically, a ruptured blood vessel in the brain.

Later that night, with a little bit of Google detective work, Mom and I find her obituary online. It is a wild sensation to see her picture on the computer screen, smiling and happy, knowing that her heart and liver are now inside me. She is gorgeous and accomplished; Mom and I get chills when we read that she had been a member of the same sorority in college that my mother, my godmother, and my sister-in-law are all a part of.

A swirling mix of gratitude and grief flows through both of us. It's a heady thing to reconcile—being alive at the expense of someone else's death. Many transplant recipients grapple with survivor's guilt and depression, and I can understand why. Having a transplant brings up all sorts of hugely existential questions and feelings:

Why am I worthy?
Why do I get to live when someone else died?

How can I possibly be deserving?

I don't have the answers to any of those questions. I don't know if there really are any answers. The best I have come up with is to try and live my life in a way that would make my donor proud. It is not uncommon for transplant recipients to have some "survivor's guilt." Though I have not much experienced guilt, per say, I do feel a huge sense of responsibility to my donors and their families.

A touch of salve is that K did not suffer, nor was there anything that would have saved her. A tragic fluke that has sparked a second chance. A second chance that I do not take lightly.

As the weeks and months pass, I settle into a nice rhythm of dialysis, work, walking, and starting to write this book. Mom, Ralph, and I get into the habit of watching a show or movie together in the evening. We play Wordle; Ralph and I watch "Family Feud" together at dinner time. We watch football in the fall and basketball in the winter and spring. It's a warm cocoon of healing and time together that would not have happened otherwise. Slight silver lining, yes?

In July of 2021, my brother and his family move forty-five minutes away. It's good for all of us to be together again. I get to enjoy an abundance of valuable family time with my mom, Ralph, my brother and his family: wife, Tiffany; my nieces, Marley, Holland, and Keller; and nephew Austin. Uncle Les and Shari. Christmases. Berry picking. Birthdays. Pool days. Outings to the local Holly Hills winery. Sushi lunch dates with Aunt Shari. Watching nieces' basketball games and seeing my nephew's basketball team win their league championship. Mornings feeding my "pet" squirrel, Diva, and our coterie of wild deer. As one famous Austinite says—LIVIN, even rockin' a dialysis port.

In May of 2021, I accept a remote adjunct position with Post University teaching an English Composition course. I also reach out to Austin Community College and begin teaching courses for them remotely, since I am still an employee. One benefit of being an adjunct is that I had simply not accepted any class assignment for the past few semesters. Now I am able to resume teaching classes online. With COVID came the huge influx of remote options, thus, I can teach from California for the time being.

In March of 2022, I am finally deemed "healthy enough" and am activated on the kidney transplant list. I immediately pack a small bag and wait. And wait. We have no way of knowing how long the wait will be, but they tell us be ready to leave for the hospital at a moment's notice.

In June 2022, Mom and Ralph travel to San Jose to attend the funeral of a close family friend, Norm Mineta, former Director of Transportation and a legendary San Jose politician. Before they leave, Mom makes me turn my phone ringer on (I always have it on silent) and we joke that, since this is the first time they have left town in a year, of course Stanford will call. I kid you not, the night before the funeral, they are getting ready for bed when my mom's phone rings. Ralph, thank God, picks up. You knew this was coming, right?

The following conversation is instantly entered into family lore. The setting: the Richards' home in Gilroy, California.

The time: 11:30 PM.

The date: Wednesday, June 15th.

Mom's phone rings while she is in the other room. Ralph answers:

Ralph: *Hello?*

Caller: *Hi, it's Eric from Stanford calling.*

Ralph: *It's a little late to be calling, don't you think?*

Caller: *I'm the kidney transplant coordinator calling for Aimee.*

Cue Ralph almost dropping the phone and running to get Mom, sputtering, "It's Stanford!"

Back home in Camino, I am turning off the lights to go to bed when the phone rings at 11:35. It's Mom. I answer and she admonishes me not picking up, saying she had called multiple times. She tells me that she has already talked to my brother and that Stanford called to say they have a kidney.

"Are you fucking kidding me!?" I scream, mostly in excitement, but partly because, of course, they would call just before midnight while Mom and Ralph are gone. Of course.

Johnny lives forty minutes away on the way to Stanford, so I call him and we decide that I will pick him up around 4:00 AM, since they want me at Stanford by 7:00 AM. I've been packed for months, but I add toiletries, then pack up my computer, phone cord, etc. I climb into bed around 1:30 AM, but it's really no use. I let my body rest, not really worrying if I fall asleep or not. A few hours later, I'm up, showered, and on the way.

I pick my brother up in the pitch-black dark and let him sleep while I drive to Stanford. I don't tell him this, but I want to drive. I want to drive myself to receive this life-changing gift. A little while later, the soft hues of sunrise start drifting delicately into the sky. Pinks and oranges streak over the highway as a few small clouds hang lazily. The Johnny Nash song about a day with bright sunshine comes to mind.

I pull up to the patient drop-off entrance and jump out, while Johnny agrees to park the car. I make my way to the wing and floor where I need to check in and approach the nurse's station.

"I'm here for a kidney transplant?" I say, more as a question than a statement, laughing at the words coming out of my mouth.

"Ah, yes! We're ready for you!" the nurse says.

I am ushered into a room, given a gown, and told surgery is scheduled for noon. My brother brings my bag to the room and hangs out with me. Soon, a nurse comes in to get a couple of IVs put in me. Mom and I text—she's getting ready for a funeral; I'm getting ready for a transplant. Nope, can't make this up.

I take a quick video update and post it to Facebook. I meet with the anesthesiologist, the coordinator, and finally the surgeon, Dr. Basque. Between "meetings," I check emails, do some grading, watch "The Price is Right." Johnny leaves after a while to get back to his family. The plan is for him to drive my car back to his house and Mom will pick it up in a day or two, then come here. Honestly, she's had enough of sitting and watching me in a hospital and this situation is night and day from two years ago. I psychically tell Dr. Chertow that I'm holding him to that *five days in and out* promise.

Shortly after noon, they roll me into the OR. The room is extremely bright and cold. It is oppressively functional-looking—not a shred of personality, but everyone is in a great mood. They get me settled with some warm blankets, talk everything over with me, and push the sleepy drugs. The next thing I know, I'm on the way to recovery.

Dr. Basque is standing over me, grinning (I can feel his smile through his mask).

"You've got a new big, beautiful kidney!" he announces.

It is the best sentence I never knew I wanted to hear.

By 7:00 PM, I am talking to my mother on the phone. Since everything went extremely well, we decide that she will come down in a couple days. I watch some TV, drink water—they now want me to drink a lot of water! When you're on dialysis, you are on fluid restrictions, so this is new. I doze off to sleep around 11:00 PM with the slightest bit of post-anesthesia fog still lingering.

A couple of days later, I am over-the-moon thrilled when Dr. Lui walks through the door. I mentally restrain myself from accosting him with a hug. We both marvel at how far I have come and how well the kidney transplant had gone. I undergo one last session of dialysis, which isn't uncommon and happens more often than not.

The kidney is doing well, but it is taking its time to "wake up," as Dr. Basque says. This is most likely due to the kidney having been on ice for an extended amount of time. Mom plays "Wake Up Little Suzie" by The Everly Brothers on her phone and we nickname the kidney "Suzie." She puts the phone on my scar and sings. If you can have fun in a hospital, we are having fun. On June 21st, she posts in the Facebook group:

When you walk in your kid's hospital room post kidney transplant that was less than 5 days ago and she's dressed in a Def Leppard shirt, dancing around and ready to go . . . so good for Momma's non-transplanted heart!!

Don't know if "Suzie" is fully awake and functioning yet. That will be determined in the days to follow with labs twice a week down here at Stanford. As soon as paperwork gets completed and all training done, we are out of here and on to Aunt Lynn & Uncle Larry's home-away-from-home!!!

While staying at Aunt Lynn and Uncle Larry's for the next few weeks, we fill the down time with mini adventures. We see the *Elvis* movie and take a couple of daytrips. Since my first surgery in 2019, I have been imploring to go to the beach, to at least just see it and smell it. So, we drive through the redwoods to Santa Cruz and right onto the pier to park. We walk the boardwalk. I buy taffy and hear the sea lions. Though I'm tempted, I decide that riding The Giant Dipper probably isn't doctor-approved quite yet. We have lunch *al fresco* with Janice, a high-school friend of Mom's. It is the definition of a sublime day.

Another day, we hit Half Moon Bay; I had scoped out a crêpe place for lunch and Mom knew a couple good spots to access the beach. Since it was still early afternoon when we finish lunch, we decide to zip over to San Francisco to do the one other thing I really wanted to do: have an Irish coffee at The Buena Vista.

The story on The Buena Vista is this: in 1952, the international travel writer, Stanton Delaplane, was at The Buena Vista. Jack Koeppler, the then-owner of The Buena Vista, challenged Delaplane to "help recreate a highly-touted Irish Coffee served at Shannon Airport in Ireland," says Buenavista.com.

After a grueling night of experimenting, with a fair amount of drinking thrown in, I'm sure, Delaplane felt defeated, but Koeppler pressed on, even traveling to Shannon Airport in Ireland! After selecting the right Irish whiskey, they still had a problem with the crème: it did not rise to the top. So, they did the next logical thing. They took the problem to a prominent local dairy owner, and mayor, of San Francisco. Finally, success! The cream settled softly at the top. And with that, an institution was born, says Buenavista.com.

This day, Mom and I are lucky enough to snag two stools at the bar, which is where you want to be if you want to see the action. The bartender, dressed in a tie and jacket, lines up eight to ten glasses at a time. First come two sugar cubes dropped into each glass. Then, he pours the scalding-hot coffee into the row of glasses in one motion going back and forth, careful to fill up each glass. A spoon is quickly plunged and swished in each glass to break up the sugar. Plunge, swish, next. Plunge, swish, next. Next, the whisky. Holding the bottle a foot and half above the glasses, he moves the bottle steadily and slowly over the glasses, again, in one motion. This is free pouring. No jiggers here. Once he reaches the end of the row, he reverses back over the row quickly, adding a little extra. Finally comes the dollop of specially-mixed cream on top. The cream is expertly, swiftly poured over the spoon, allowing for a gorgeous, one-inch-thick float. It's hard not to be mesmerized by the process. It's my theory that the process is part of what makes it taste so good. This day, it tastes like hard-earned victory.

One of my favorite post-transplant pictures is from this day. Me, sitting at that bar wearing a sweatshirt gifted to me by Mom that says, "Note to Self: You Are Doing Great." Irish coffee in hand. No IVs. No trach. No dialysis port. My hair has, after a year, come back in. I look healthy. I look happy. I *am* happy. I look and feel whole.

After Buena Vista, we hit up Ghirardelli Chocolate, because, if you're going to have a splurge day, why not go all out? We get ice cream and snag one of the small tables for two as a throng of people are out enjoying the day. I email a few pictures to Dr. Lui, Dr. Vagelos, and Dr. MacArthur.

I'm told ice cream and Irish coffee are medicinal, right? I write.

You are an inspiration and ice cream is definitely therapeutic! writes Dr. Lui.

You are the hero in this adventure! writes Dr. Vagelos.

After a month, we return home to Camino as everything continues to go well. The scar—this rough, pink, lopsided smile on the left side of my midsection—heals nicely.

Upon my follow-up clinic visit a month later, the nephrologist, Dr. Ahern, says I'm doing so well that he doesn't need to see me in person for another two months, and suggests a video visit in the meantime for a month from now. When I return for a clinic visit at the six-month mark with zero complications, the doctor, Mom, and I look at each other.

"You're doing so well, Aimee . . . I've got nothing," Dr. Ahearn says. Our laugh says what isn't being said: *It's been hell, but we've made it!*

Indeed, "I've got nothing" is music to all of our ears and not something Mom and I are used to hearing from a doctor. We float out of the visit on a cloud of *Hell Yeah!* and stop at a Shake Shack next to the hospital for lunch before driving home. One definition of the word "nothing" is *the absence of all magnitude or quantity.* For years, we have been working toward and hoping for this *nothing.* We sit down and eat, basking in the glow of that *nothing.*

So, what do you do when you've finally clawed your life back from hell?

NINETEEN

IN NOVEMBER 2022 WITH MY DOCTORS' PERMISSION, I take my long-awaited first airplane ride since 2019 to visit Dad in Las Vegas. To say that I've missed traveling is a gross understatement. We go to the Mob Museum, located in an old, converted courthouse. We watch a short film about famous mob cases that took place in that actual courtroom in the courthouse. We participate in a Cirque Du Soleil show called "Mad Apple." We eat delicious food and have some superb wine. We have a ball and I am beyond excited to be able to travel again.

So much so that in December, I take a trip to Austin, Texas, mostly to visit friends, and to attend a poetry reading organized by two good poet friends, Jim and Christia. I spend a week soaking in the love and friendships: Happy hour at Eddie V's steakhouse, a visit to the Museum of Ice Cream, wine and girl talk, and going to the *Elf* movie party at the Alamo Drafthouse. My friend Janiece and I started going to the *Elf* movie party years ago and it turned into an annual event, complete with Christmas light necklaces and Santa hats. I am psyched to be able to go again! It is a perfect holiday Austin visit.

Fast forward to June 2023. I move back to Austin, Texas. After feeling like I had my life pulled out from under me at the end of 2019, it feels right and necessary to return. I am not done with Austin. And I don't think it's done with me, yet, either.

I move into my friend Erica's two bedroom/two-bathroom apartment. Since we are both in our forties, we decide that the only logical way to decorate is with squirrels and unicorns, as a nod to her obsession with squirrels (she is a squirrel rehabber) and my fondness for unicorns and the Team Glitter Unicorn Facebook page. I find a small, wooden sign on Etsy that says, "Welcome to the Nuthouse," with a graphic of a squirrel and some acorns. We dub the place the Nuthouse.

I buy a new bed and dresser, along with a shower curtain that says, "Paris is always a good idea." I unpack three years' worth of life that had been lovingly packed away. I hang posters and pictures and fill three small bookshelves. I even find the cutest small painting of a squirrel holding a glass of wine and wearing pearls. Naming her Dorothy Parker as a nod to one of my earliest literary heroes, I hang her above the kitchen sink next to the sign. She is sweet and sassy looking. Just like Erica and me. Though Mom's place has been—and is—a heaven on earth, it's empowering and regenerative to have a bit of my own space again. New parts. Fresh start.

✳

I have been asked a few times what it's like having transplanted organs.

Do my insides "feel different"? No. There are stories of transplant patients who have taken on traits or had "memories" from their donor, such as Claire Sylvia, a forty-year-old former ballet dancer who received the heart of an eighteen-year-old male and suddenly found herself craving Kentucky Fried Chicken and beer, according to a *Psychology Today* article by Thomas R. Vernay, MD, called, "Heart Transplants, Personality Transplants?"[13] (Verney).

I have not experienced such phenomena, but I do find it fascinating. For better or worse, I still seem to be the same

Paris/Prince/purple-obsessed, bookworm poet that I always was. Still me, just some recycled parts.

It is strange to know that you have someone else's organs. It is a wild and inescapable fact that is never out of my peripheral thoughts. I constantly think about my donors, their families, my doctors, and my nurses. After my transplant, Mom would sometimes call me Aimee 2.0. I never liked drawing attention to or talking about my heart defect much before, and I feel mostly the same way about my transplants. It doesn't define me, but, at the same time, it would be a huge disservice not to acknowledge this life-giving and scientifically miraculous gift.

When I visited the J-Wing of Stanford almost two years after my heart and liver transplant, one of the nurses, Monica, who had been there throughout, asked me if I would do the whole thing over again, knowing how tough it had been.

A thousand. Fucking. Percent.

PHOTO GALLERY

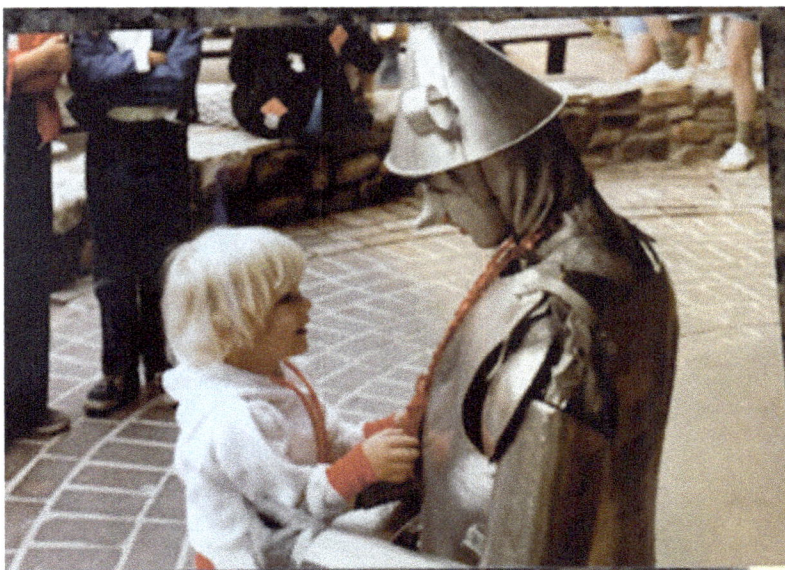

Aimee with the Tin Man at Land of Oz. 1979-80.

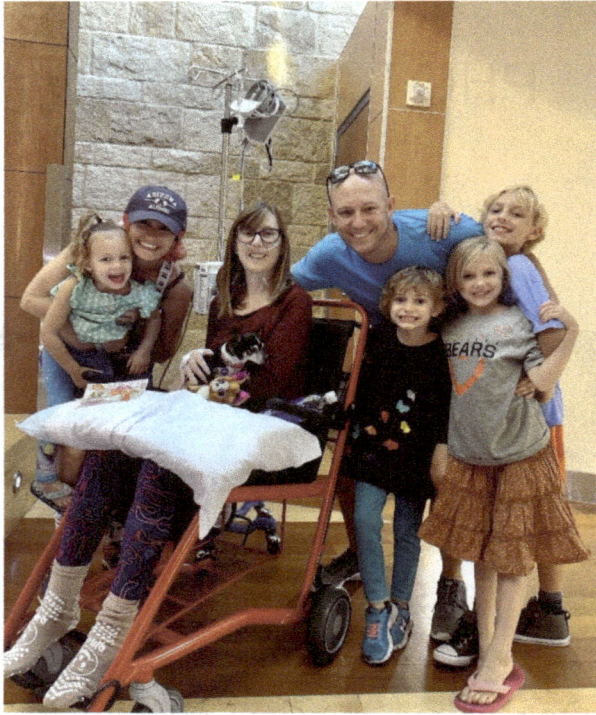

Family smuggling in Elphie to Dell hospital. October 2019.

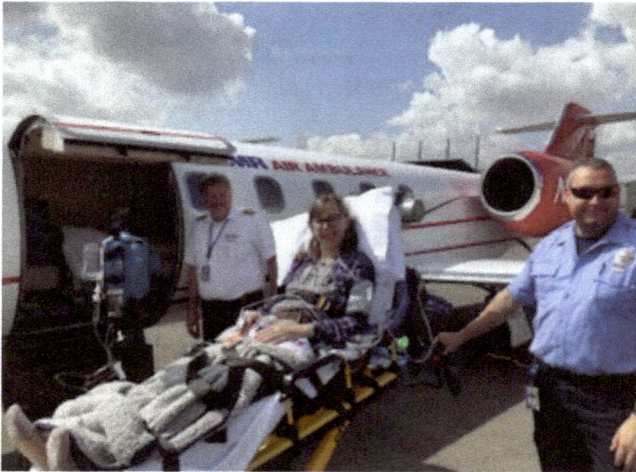

October 9th, 2019. Flying to Stanford.

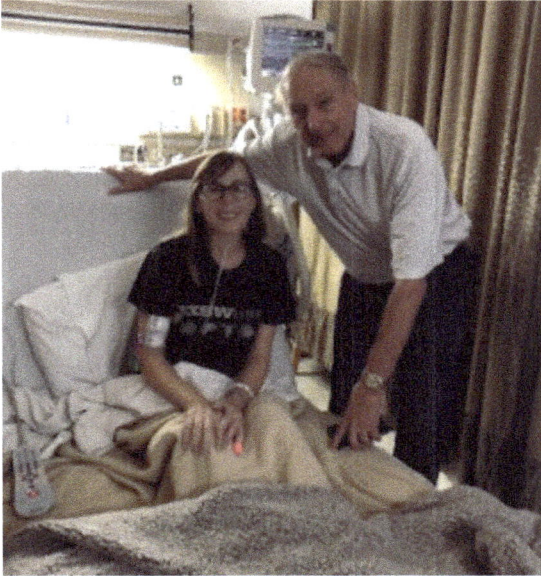

Aimee & Dad. October 14th, 2019.

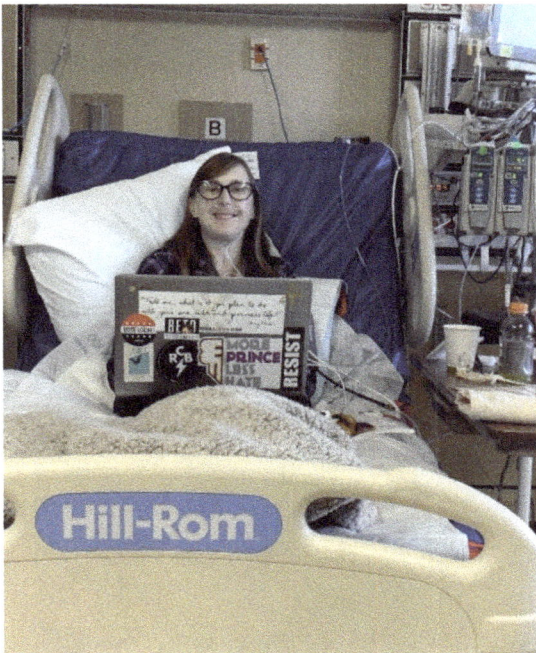

Working. October 2019.

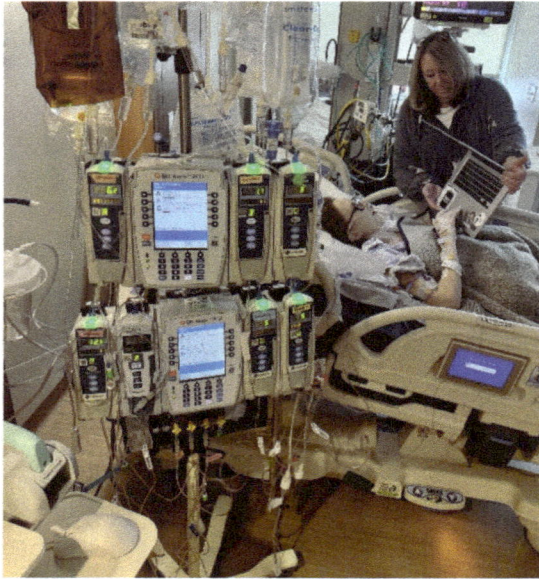

Mom holding up my computer so I can write to my jobs before going into ECMO surgery. Thanksgiving 2019.

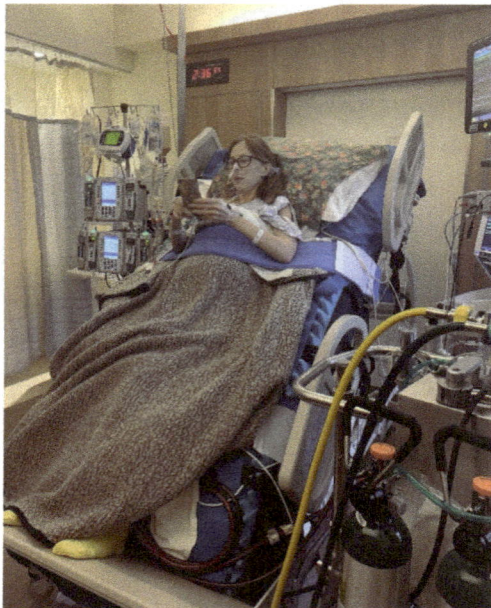

Chillin' on ECMO. December 3rd, 2019.

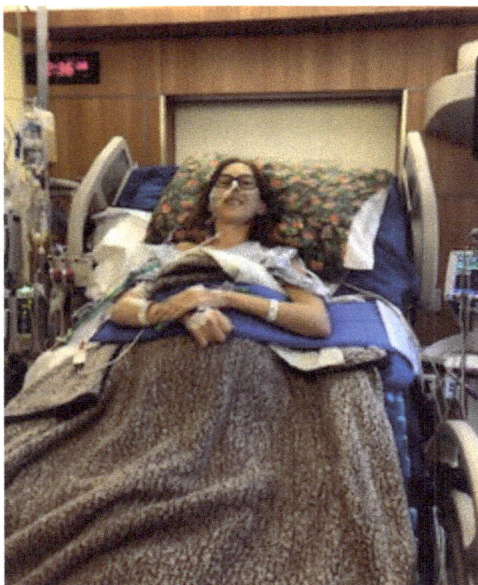

Waiting for a heart and liver. December 3rd, 2019.

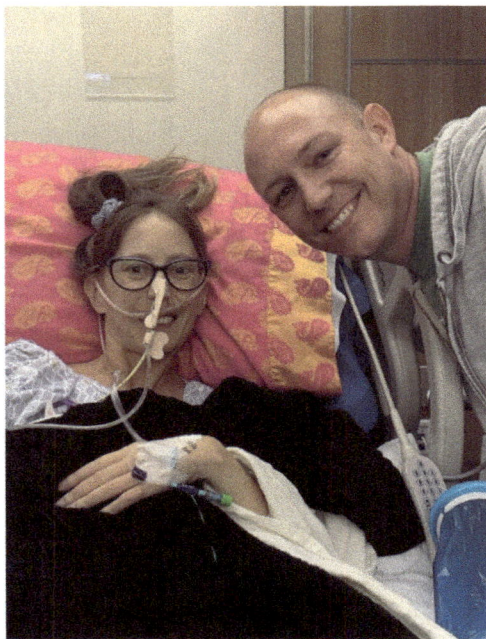

Johnny visits. December 6th, 2019.

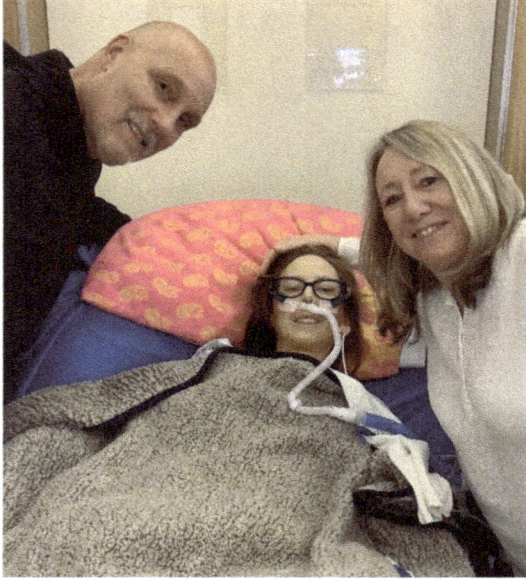

Ralph, Aimee, & Mom before being taken off to surgery. December 12th, 2019.

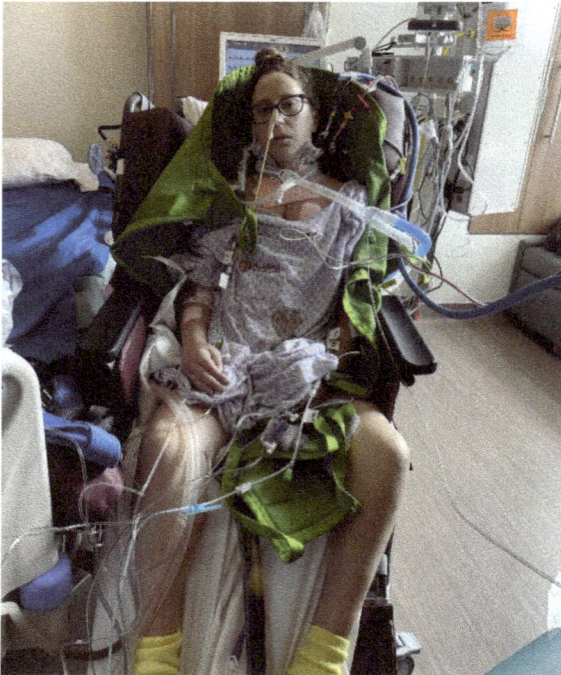

Twelve days post-surgery. Christmas 2019.

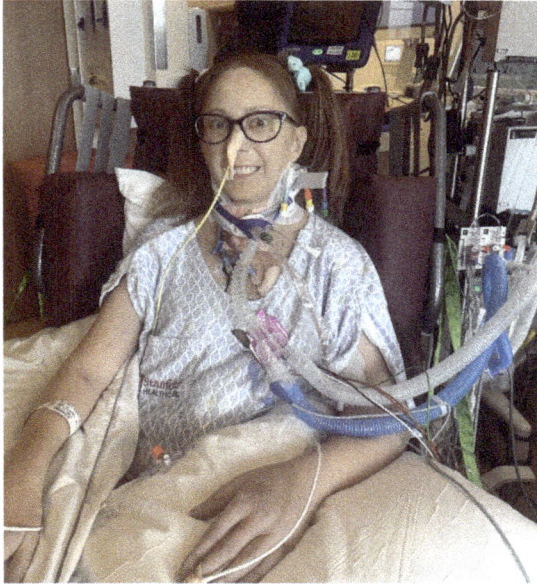

January 5th, 2020.

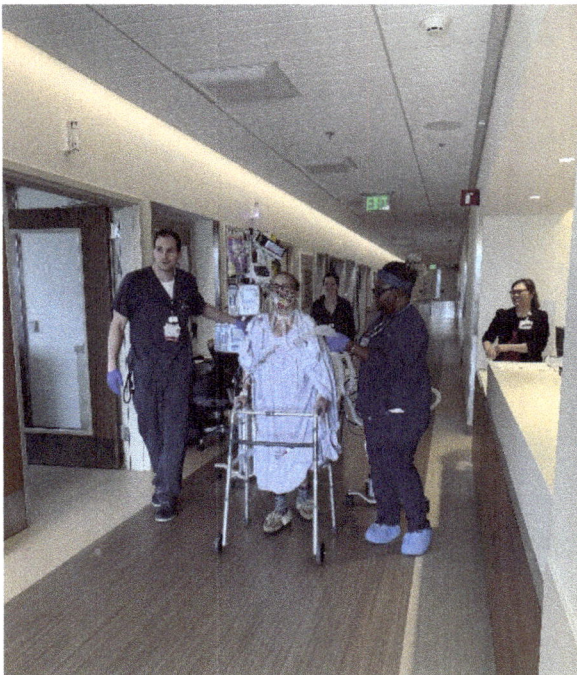

Walking. February 16th, 2020.

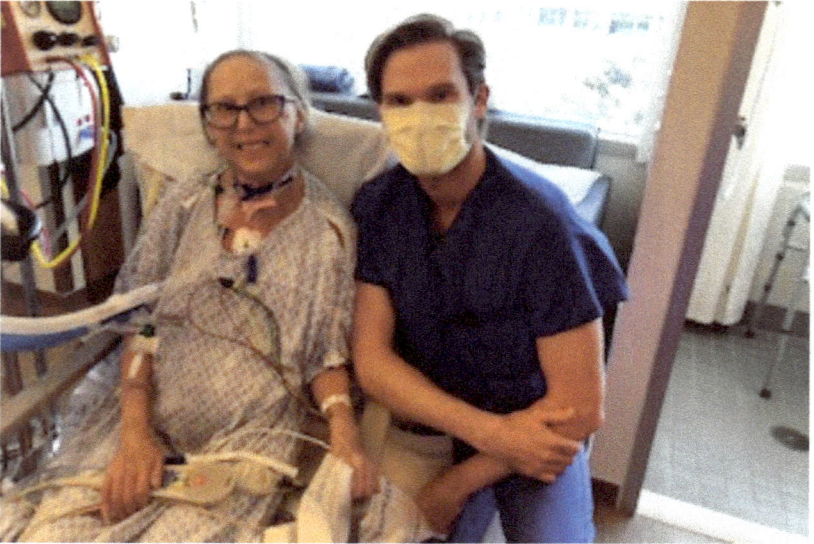

Aimee & Dr. J.W. MacArthur. June 16th. Day of transport to Kentfield.

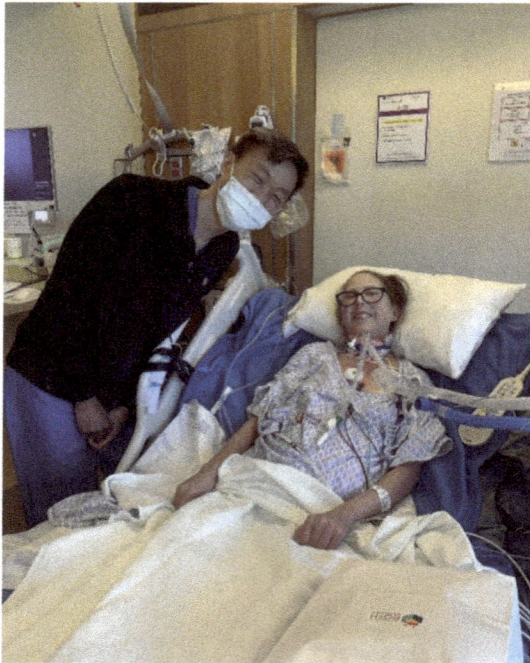

Aimee & Dr. George Lui. June 16th. Day of transport to Kentfield.

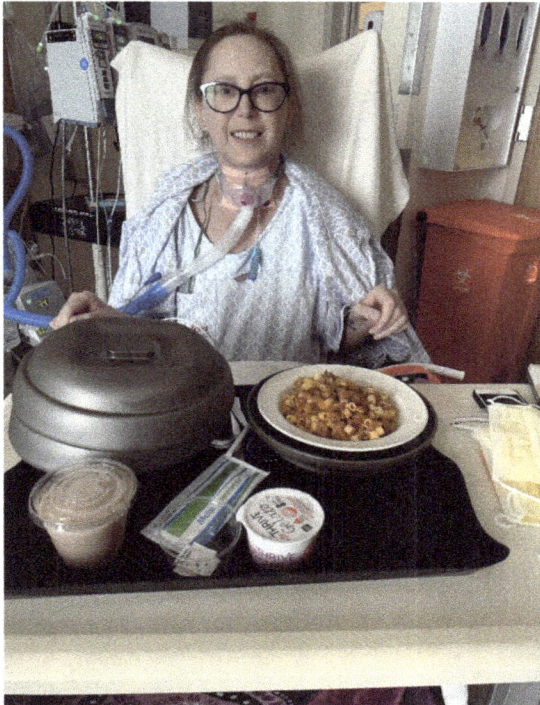

Solid foods! August 13th, 2020.

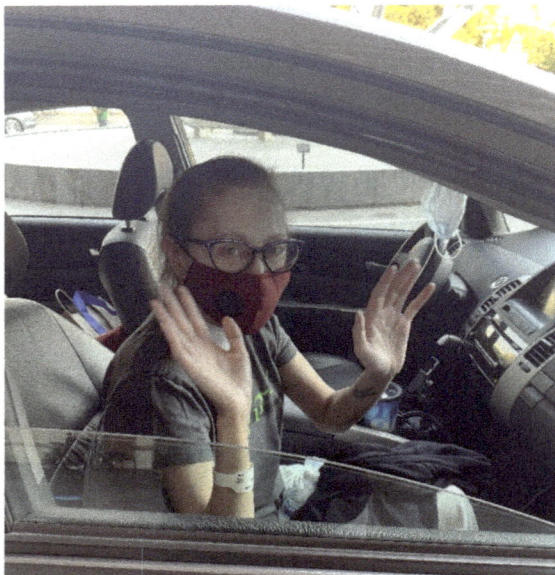

Going Home! August 25th, 2020.

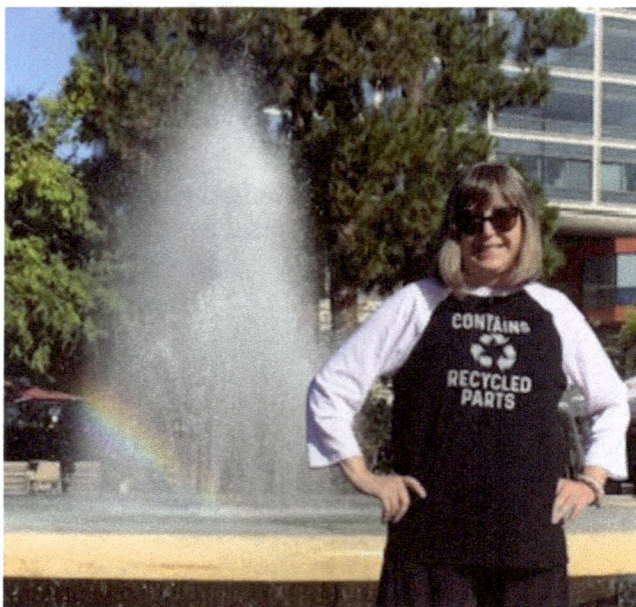

August 2022. Triple transplant level unlocked.

ACKNOWLEDGMENTS & THANKS

TO MY DONORS' FAMILIES: "THANK YOU" IS NOT enough to express my gratitude to your loved ones' life-saving selflessness. It is an honor to hold a bit of them with me. I hope to make you all proud every day.

Unmeasurable love and gratitude to Dr. George Lui, Dr. Randall Vagelos, and Dr. J.W. MacArthur and teams for saving my life more than once and in more than one way. I am forever your servant.

A huge hug and thank you to Dr. Charles Fraser for absolutely everything. To the best nurses and staff at Stanford: Dorothy, Bridgitte, Monica, Leah, Jake, Adam, Ben, Mara, Rangel, Karen, Sarah, Julia, Samantha, and so many others. Thank you, thank you, thank you! My family and I think of all of you all the time.

To Aunt Lynn and Uncle Larry, love and thanks for the use of your house and the lasagna and fruit tarts.

To my friends, family, and Team Glitter Unicorn, your love and support were as much a part of my recovery as anything. Thank you for your love, the gifts, and your endless support of our family. It is felt and treasured.

To Elizabeth Ann Atkins at Two Sisters Writing & Publishing®, thank you for coaching me, then editing and publishing this book, along with all the encouragement and praise to help me make this book dream come true.

To Janiece and Erica, thank you for your love, support and help with my move back to Austin. To Johnny and Tiffany, eternal love, thanks, and gratitude for dropping everything to move me out of my apartment within a week, for basically taking over my life when I was in the hospital, and for so much more.

To Dad, thank you for your endless love, moral support, daily affirmation emails, and financial support. To Mom and Ralph, thank you for all your love, caring, the guest room that came with deer and squirrels, and cooking over the past three years.

To Ralph, my bonus Dad, to being here every step of the way and many, many rides to dialysis. I could not have done it without you.

And to Mom, additionally, for saving my life multiple times.

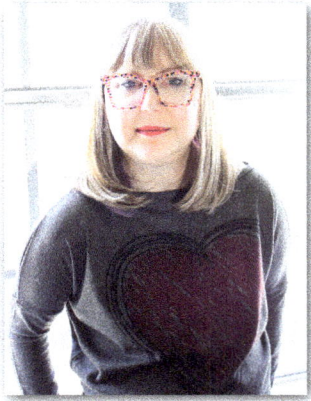

AUTHOR BIO

AIMEE MACKOVIC IS ALIVE BECAUSE OF TWO selfless donors. She is an award-winning poet, writer of creative non-fiction, and professor of English who works and writes from Austin, Texas.

She graduated with her B.A from Wake Forest University and her M.F.A. from Spalding University. Before she began teaching, she worked in costume shops in New York City making costumes for Broadway.

Her books of poetry include *Headlines* (dancing girl press, 2023), *Love Junky* (Lit City Press, 2017), and *A Sentenced Woman* (Finishing Line Press, 2007).

Find her at aimeemackovic.com.

ENDNOTES

[1] White, Tracie. "The First U.S. Adult Heart Transplant." Stanford Medicine Magazine, 26 Feb. 2018, stanmed.stanford.edu/fifty-years-since-first-us-adult-heart-transplant-stanford/.

[2] White, Tracie. "The First U.S. Adult Heart Transplant." *Stanford Medicine Magazine*, 26 Feb. 2018, stanmed.stanford.edu/fifty-years-since-first-us-adult-heart-transplant-stanford/.

[3] White, Tracie. "The First U.S. Adult Heart Transplant." *Stanford Medicine Magazine*, 26 Feb. 2018, stanmed.stanford.edu/fifty-years-since-first-us-adult-heart-transplant-stanford/.

[4] "Heart Transplant Sets All-Time Record in 2021." *UNOS*, 17 Feb. 2022, unos.org/news/in-focus/heart-transplant-all-time-record-2021. Accessed 13 July 2023.

[5] Hemmati, Pouya, et al. "One Hundred and Counting: Dr Dwight C. McGoon's Enduring Legacy." *The Annals of Thoracic Surgery*, vol. 108, no. 2, Aug. 2019, pp. 641–644, https://doi.org/10.1016/j.athoracsur.2019.02.073. Accessed 13 Nov. 2021.

[6] Hemmati, Pouya, et al. "One Hundred and Counting: Dr Dwight C. McGoon's Enduring Legacy." *The Annals of Thoracic Surgery*, vol. 108, no. 2, Aug. 2019, pp. 641–644, https://doi.org/10.1016/j.athoracsur.2019.02.073. Accessed 13 Nov. 2021.

[7] "Turner Syndrome – Symptoms and Causes." *Mayo Clinic*, Mayo Clinic, 18 Nov. 2017, www.mayoclinic.org/diseases-conditions/turner-syndrome/symptoms-causes/syc-20360782.

[8] "Unicorn | Mythological Creature." *Encyclopedia Britannica*, 24 May 2018, www.britannica.com/topic/unicorn. Accessed 7 June 2023.

[9] Kim, JL, et al. "Extracorporeal Membrane Oxygenator as a Bridge to Heart-Liver En Bloc Transplant in a Fontan Patient,." *JTCVS Techniques*, 2022, https://doi.org/10.1016/j.xjtc.2022.01.018.

[10] Fabrizi F, Dixit V, Martin P, Messa P. Chronic kidney disease after liver transplantation: Recent evidence. Int J Artif Organs. 2010 Nov;33(11):803-11. PMID: 21140356, https://pubmed.ncbi.nlm.nih.gov/21140356/

[11] Vaish, A., Grossmann, T., & Woodward, A. (2008). Not all emotions are created equal: The negativity bias in social-emotional development. *Psychological Bulletin, 134*(3), 383–403. http://doi.org/10.1037/0033-2909.134.383

[12] Chowdhury, Madhuleena Roy. "The Neuroscience of Gratitude and How It Affects Anxiety & Grief." *PositivePsychology.com*, 9 Apr. 2019, positivepsychology.com/neuroscience-of-gratitude/.

[13] Vernay, Thomas R. MD. "Heart Transplants, Personality Transplants?" Psychology Today, 21 October 2021, https://www.psychologytoday.com/us/blog/explorations-the-mind/202110/heart-transplants-personality-transplants